60 HIKES
WITHIN 60 MILES

ATLANTA
INCLUDING
MARIETTA, LAWRENCEVILLE, AND PEACHTREE CITY

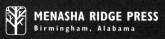

MENASHA RIDGE PRESS
Birmingham, Alabama

60 HIKES WITHIN 60 MILES

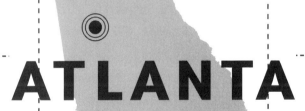

ATLANTA

INCLUDING
**Marietta,
Lawrenceville,
and Peachtree City**

SECOND EDITION

RANDY AND PAM GOLDEN

DISCLAIMER

This book is meant only as a guide to select trails in the Atlanta area and does not guarantee hiker safety in any way—you hike at your own risk. Neither Menasha Ridge Press nor Randy or Pam Golden is liable for property loss or damage, personal injury, or death that result in any way from accessing or hiking the trails described in the following pages. Please be aware that hikers have been injured in the Atlanta area. Be especially cautious when walking on or near boulders, steep inclines, and drop-offs, and do not attempt to explore terrain that may be beyond your abilities. To help ensure an uneventful hike, please read carefully the introduction to this book, and perhaps get further safety information and guidance from other sources. Familiarize yourself thoroughly with the areas you intend to visit before venturing out. Ask questions, and prepare for the unforeseen. Familiarize yourself with current weather reports, maps of the area you intend to visit, and any relevant park regulations.

Copyright 2008 Randy and Pam Golden
All rights reserved
Printed in the United States of America
Published by Menasha Ridge Press
Distributed by Publishers Group West
Second edition, first printing

Library of Congress Cataloging-in-Publication Data
Golden, Randy, 1953-
60 hikes within 60 miles : Atlanta, including Marietta, Lawrenceville, and Peachtree
City / by Randy and Pam Golden. -- 2nd ed.
    p. cm.
 Includes bibliographical references and index.
 ISBN-13: 978-0-89732-673-5 (alk. paper)
 ISBN-10: 0-89732-673-3 (alk. paper)
 1. Hiking--Georgia--Atlanta Region--Guidebooks. 2. Atlanta Region (Ga.)--Guide-
books. I. Golden, Pam. II. Title. III. Title: Sixty hikes within sixty miles.

GV199.42.G462A855 2008
917.5804'44--dc22

                          2008020896

Cover design by Steveco International and Scott McGrew
Text design by Steveco International
Cover photo by Pam Golden
Author photo by Pam Golden
All other photos by Randy and Pam Golden
Maps by Scott McGrew and Randy Golden

Menasha Ridge Press
PO. Box 43673
Birmingham, AL 35243
www.menasharidge.com

TABLE OF CONTENTS

ACKNOWLEDGMENTS

First and foremost, Pam and I want to thank the dedicated individuals whose hard work created and maintains these trails. Without them this book would not be possible. Additionally, we owe a debt of gratitude to the scores of park rangers who freely shared their time and knowledge of their area's history, flora and fauna, and interesting trivia.

There are many other people who made a significant contribution, including Steve Storey, an outdoor enthusiast who works for the State of Georgia and gave us a number of ideas for hikes to include in the book. Finally, a heartfelt thanks goes to the folks at Menasha Ridge Press, especially Russell Helms, who patiently guided us throughout this adventure.

—RANDY GOLDEN

FOREWORD

Welcome to Menasha Ridge Press's *60 Hikes within 60 Miles,* a series designed to provide hikers with information needed to find and hike the very best trails surrounding cities usually underserved by good guidebooks.

Our strategy was simple: First, find a hiker who knows the area and loves to hike. Second, ask that person to spend a year researching the most popular and very best trails around. And third, have that person describe each trail in terms of difficulty, scenery, condition, elevation change, and all other categories of information that are important to hikers. "Pretend you've just completed a hike and met up with other hikers at the trailhead," we told each author. "Imagine their questions; be clear in your answers."

Experienced hikers and writers, authors Randy and Pam Golden have selected 60 of the best hikes in and around the Atlanta metropolitan area. From the greenways and urban hikes that highlight Atlanta's diverse population to flora- and fauna-rich treks amid state and national parks in the hinterlands, the Goldens provide hikers (and walkers) with a great variety of hikes—and all within roughly 60 miles of Atlanta.

You'll get more out of this book if you take a moment to read the Introduction explaining how to use the trail profiles. The Topographic Maps section will help you understand how useful topos will be on a hike and will also tell you where to get them. And though this is a "where-to," not a "how-to" guide, those of you who have not hiked extensively will find the Introduction of particular value.

As much for the opportunity to free the spirit as to free the body, let these hikes elevate you above the urban melee.

All the best,
The Editors at Menasha Ridge Press

ABOUT THE AUTHORS

Randy and Pam Golden have shared their lifelong love of hiking since they met at college in Florida in 1975. After marrying in 1977, they began hiking across the United States and into Canada. Among their favorite foreign destinations are Puerto

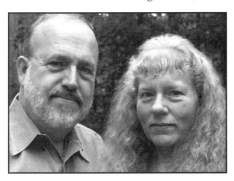

Rico's El Yunque and Australia's Dandenong Mountains. They began writing about their adventures on About North Georgia (**www.ngeorgia.com**) in 1995. In 1998 the site's Trails section was spun off into a site of its own, Georgia Trails (**www.georgiatrails.com**).

PREFACE

As Pam and I told folks about our venture, writing *60 Hikes Within 60 Miles*, we frequently heard, "There are 60 trails in the Atlanta area?" Our problem was not finding trails but deciding which ones best represented the tremendous variety available. In addition to Lawrenceville, Marietta, and Peachtree City, our area included a portion of the Georgia mountains—a well-known hiking destination—and hiking-oriented towns like Roswell and Cartersville. The hardest place to find representative trails was south of the city, but that is changing: Great additions like Sprewell Bluff, a Georgia state park, Charlie Elliot, and Cochran Mill have increased the number of hiking trails available there.

ATLANTA: AMERICA'S FIRST GREAT INLAND CITY

According to tradition, Stephen Long rode a horse to Hardy Ivy's cabin, placed a marker at the site of the 0 mile post of the Western and Atlantic Railroad, and then returned to his office in Marietta. Although Long did not really place the marker at what today is the heart of downtown Atlanta, he did write in his journal that the area would never amount to much. Even the man charged with building the railroad did not understand the importance of this revolutionary mode of transportation.

Farmers and businessmen, though, quickly learned, and by the time the Western and Atlantic was completed in 1850, Atlanta was a thriving rail hub that had already undergone two name changes (Terminus and Marthasville). Formerly a hard ride of two days (or more, depending on what you were carrying), Chattanooga was now just ten hours away by train, traveling at the astounding speed of 10 miles per hour. Soon it became apparent that for a railroad to survive, it had to come to Atlanta.

Unscathed by the Civil War until 1864, the railroads brought Atlanta its utter destruction. Union general William Tecumseh Sherman followed the Western and Atlantic to Atlanta, where he earned two sobriquets, "the father of modern warfare" and "the father of urban renewal." He ordered the central city burned before leaving it. With less than two dollars in the city treasury, Atlanta began to rebuild.

Opportunity in the burgeoning city attracted a wide variety of people, including former slaves. The freemen formed a community centered around the African American churches on Auburn Avenue, just east of downtown. John Wesley Dobbs anointed the town "Sweet Auburn" and, referencing economic development, proclaimed the streets "paved with gold." The community formed the nucleus of the civil rights movement in the South and was the birthplace of many of the movement's early leaders, including Martin Luther King Jr. Sadly, with each door opened by the integration of Atlanta, one closed on Sweet Auburn. But the district began to revive in the 1990s.

Farmers and farmhands were attracted to higher-paying industrial jobs in the growing city, and what was a trickle of new people at the start of the 20th century became a flood in the 1920s, helped by the boll weevil, falling cotton prices, and a historic drought. Well-to-do Atlantans moved north to Ansley Park and Druid Hills. When airplanes began to take over mail routes from the railroads, Atlanta built an airport to once again become a hub in southeastern transportation. Although the first airmail route, between Atlanta and Miami, lasted less than a year, more followed, and by 1930 planes were a common sight in the skies over the capital of the Peach State.

After trying for many years, in the 1960s Atlanta became a Major League town with its Braves and Falcons and later the Hawks and Thrashers. Jimmy Carter built the first Presidential Library here amid much controversy, and a memorial to Dr. King and the civil rights movement was completed in the 1980s. In 1996 Atlanta hosted the Summer Olympics, building Centennial Park in a blighted area of downtown, now the site of Georgia Aquarium and the World of Coca-Cola.

THE TRAILS

The trails in this book are a diverse combination of hikes in terms of location, type of hike, and length, but there are a couple of distinct areas where there is some concentration of trails. The largest number of trails is in the Chattahoochee River National Recreation Area. Other sites with multiple trails are Georgia's state park system, which has hiking opportunities throughout the area; the Chattahoochee National Forest, which forms the northern rim of the designated area; and Kennesaw Mountain National Battlefield Park, designed to memorialize the men who fought and died in the bloodiest battle of the Atlanta Campaign and at other Civil War sites.

CHATTAHOOCHEE RIVER NATIONAL RECREATION AREA

In 1978 President Jimmy Carter signed into law a bill creating the Chattahoochee River National Recreation Area (CRNRA). It encompasses 16 named parks (currently totaling 9,271 acres), although some of the parks are designated for future development. They are designed to offer a wide range of outdoor fun, including hiking, biking, walking, canoeing, kayaking, and rafting. The park's headquarters is at the Island Ford Unit, where you can buy a season pass to all the units for $25. Otherwise, each visit will cost you $3, paid at the trail kiosk in the parking lots. The most popular park in the system is Cochran Shoals, just north of Interstate 285. The most scenic is East Palisades, and the most remote is Bowman's Island, just south of Lake Lanier. Fulton County, Cobb County, Gwinnett County, and Forsyth County each have park areas within the boundaries of the CRNRA.

Although not part of the national recreation area, the Chattahoochee Nature Center is adjacent to the river and offers a good hike along with informative displays and creatures from the wild. There is an extensive area of raptors, including two American bald eagles.

The river flows northwest of downtown Atlanta, and there are some great places not far off its route to stay, eat, and sleep, including Cobb County's Cumberland Mall/Galleria area, Sandy Springs, and Roswell, in Fulton County.

CHATTAHOOCHEE NATIONAL FOREST

The northern rim of our 60-mile area is covered by the Chattahoochee National Forest. Originally part of the Cherokee National Forest, the area was reorganized along state lines in the 1930s, and the Chattahoochee National Forest was created. Within its bounds are Georgia's high point, Brasstown Bald, and the unusually named Blood Mountain, which was the site of a battle between the area's earlier inhabitants, Creek and Cherokee natives. There are hundreds of hikes in this national forest, most of which are outside the 60-mile radius from Atlanta. We have chosen three that represent why we love the Georgia mountains.

If you are intrigued by our choices and would like to continue your exploration, we recommend Tim Homan's excellent book, *The Hiking Trails of North Georgia*. Unlike the sharp, tall peaks farther north in the Appalachian Mountains, Georgia's Blue Ridge Mountains are somewhat softer but are not "easy," in any sense of the word. The remote nature of these mountain trails makes them great for solitude, but be careful—if you are injured on a hike, it will be difficult to contact rescue personnel, much less get them to your location. We don't want you to be afraid of hiking in the mountains; we have been doing it for years. Just follow a few obvious safety tips: Don't hike in the mountains alone, make sure somebody knows exactly where you are going and when you will be back, be cautious of wildlife management areas during hunting season, and bring a map and compass, even if you have a GPS receiver.

When you are done traipsing through the woods, Georgia's mountain towns have some good dining to offer. In Blue Ridge (the city, not the mountain range), check out The Cabin Grill, Colonel Poole's BBQ in Ellijay, or for expansive family dining, Smith House in Dahlonega and the Dillard House north of Clayton. Excellent accommodations greatly improve the hike. Enota, near Brasstown Bald, is our favorite for a cabin/camping experience, or, for an upscale resort, try Brasstown Valley or Fieldstone Inn.

GEORGIA'S STATE PARKS

One of the best things about Georgia is the state parks. They combine a huge array of entertainment, and we don't mean just hiking. From Stone Mountain, where the fun is practically endless, to the highest falls east of the Mississippi (Amicalola), and the only capital city of the Cherokee Nation in the eastern United States (New Echota), Georgia's state parks form a nucleus of excellent hiking and other fun pursuits. Other state parks whose hiking trails are included in the book are Sprewell Bluff, Pickett's Mill, High Falls, Sweetwater, and Hard Labor Creek.

KENNESAW MOUNTAIN NATIONAL BATTLEFIELD PARK
AND OTHER CIVIL WAR SITES

When Ulysses S. Grant took over command of the Union Army in 1864, he initiated a coordinated effort to end the Confederacy. While the Army of the Potomac marched against Robert E. Lee and his Army of Northern Virginia, Sherman marched against Joe Johnston's Army of Tennessee, which defended Georgia. Sherman engaged the Rebels at Dalton, Resaca, New Hope Church, Pickett's Mill, Dallas, Kolb's Farm, Kennesaw Mountain, Peachtree Creek, Atlanta, Ezra Church, and Jonesboro before claiming the city of Atlanta as "ours, and fairly won." In the middle of these battles, Confederate president Jefferson Davis replaced Johnston with John B. Hood, a more aggressive but less capable general. Following the loss of Atlanta, Hood moved into north Georgia, where he engaged Union forces at Allatoona Pass before moving north into Tennessee.

Hikes that visit battlefields include Pickett's Mill; Kolb's Farm, Burnt Hickory Loop, and Cheatham Hill (Kennesaw Mountain); Miss Daisy's Atlanta (Freedom Parkway passes through the site of Confederate and Union lines; the site of Sherman's headquarters during the Battle of Atlanta is at the Carter Center); and Allatoona Pass.

HIKING RECOMMENDATIONS

HIKES GOOD FOR CHILDREN *(continued)*

HIKES GOOD FOR SOLITUDE

HIKES GOOD FOR WILDLIFE VIEWING

HIKES WITH STEEP SECTIONS

HISTORIC TRAILS

HISTORIC TRAILS *(continued)*

LAKE HIKES

SCENIC HIKES

TRAILS GOOD FOR MOUNTAIN BIKES

TRAILS GOOD FOR RUNNERS

TRAILS GOOD FOR RUNNERS *(continued)*

URBAN HIKES

HIKES LESS THAN 3 MILES

HIKES 3 TO 6 MILES

HIKES 3 TO 6 MILES (continued)

HIKES LONGER THAN 6 MILES

INTRODUCTION

Welcome to *60 Hikes within 60 Miles: Atlanta.* If you're new to hiking or even if you're a seasoned trail-smith, take a few minutes to read the following introduction. We explain how this book is organized and how to use it.

HOW TO USE THIS GUIDEBOOK

THE OVERVIEW MAP AND OVERVIEW MAP KEY

Use the overview map on the inside front cover to assess the exact locations of each hike's primary trailhead. Each hike's number appears on the overview map, on the map key facing the overview map, and in the table of contents. As you flip through the book, a hike's full profile is easy to locate by watching for the hike number at the top of each page. The book is organized by region as indicated in the table of contents. A map legend that details the symbols found on trail maps appears on the inside back cover.

REGIONAL MAPS

The book is divided into regions, and prefacing each regional section is an overview map of that region. The regional map provides more detail than the overview map, bringing you closer to the hike.

TRAIL MAPS

Each hike contains a detailed map that shows the trailhead, the route, significant features, facilities, and topographic landmarks such as creeks, overlooks, and peaks. The authors gathered map data by carrying a Garmin eTrex Legend GPS unit while hiking. This data was downloaded into a digital mapping program (Delorme) and processed by expert cartographers to produce the highly accurate maps found in this book. Each trailhead's GPS coordinates are included with each profile.

ELEVATION PROFILES

Corresponding directly to the trail map, each hike contains a detailed elevation profile. The elevation profile provides a quick look at the trail from the side, enabling you to visualize how the trail rises and falls. Key points along the way are labeled. Note the number of feet between each tick mark on the vertical axis (the height scale). To avoid making flat hikes look steep and steep hikes appear flat, height scales are used throughout the book to provide an accurate image of the hike's climbing difficulty.

GPS TRAILHEAD COORDINATES

To collect accurate map data, each trail was hiked with a handheld GPS unit (Garmin eTrexseries). Data collected was then downloaded and plotted onto a digital USGS topo map. In addition to rendering a highly specific trail outline, this book also includes the GPS coordinates for each trailhead in two formats: latitude/longitude and UTM. Latitude/longitude coordinates tell you where you are by locating a point west (latitude) of the 0° meridian line that passes through Greenwich, England, and north or south of the 0° (longitude) line that belts the Earth, a.k.a. the equator.

Topographic maps show latitude/longitude as well as UTM grid lines. Known as UTM coordinates, the numbers index a specific point using a grid method. The survey datum used to arrive at the coordinates in this book is NAD27 (versus WGS84 or WGS83). For readers who own a GPS unit, whether handheld or onboard a vehicle, the latitude/longitude or UTM coordinates provided on the first page of each hike may be entered into the GPS unit. Just make sure your GPS unit is set to navigate using NAD27 datum. Now you can navigate directly to the trailhead.

Most trailheads, which begin in parking areas, can be reached by car, but some hikes still require a short walk to reach the trailhead from a parking area. In those cases a handheld unit is necessary to continue the GPS navigation process. However, readers can easily access all trailheads in this book by using the directions given, the overview map, and the trail map, which shows at least one major road leading into the area. But for those who enjoy using the latest GPS technology to navigate, the necessary data has been provided. Here is an example from Arabia Mountain on page 212:

UTM Zone (NAD27)	**16S**
Easting	**0766670**
Northing	**3727921**

The UTM zone number (16) refers to one of the 60 vertical zones of the Universal Transverse Mercator (UTM) projection. Each zone is 6 degrees wide. The UTM zone letter (S) refers to one of the 20 horizontal zones that span from 80 degrees south to 84 degrees north. The easting number (0766670 indicates in meters how far east or west a point is from the central meridian of the zone.

Increasing easting coordinates on a topo map or on your GPS screen indicate that you are moving east; decreasing easting coordinates indicate you are moving west. The northing number (3727921) references in meters how far you are from the equator. Above and below the equator, increasing northing coordinates indicate you are traveling north; decreasing northing coordinates indicate you are traveling south. To learn more about how to enhance your outdoor experiences with GPS technology, refer to *GPS Outdoors: A Practical Guide for Outdoor Enthusiasts* (Menasha Ridge Press).

HIKE DESCRIPTIONS

Each hike contains seven key items: an "In Brief" description of the trail, a key at-a-glance box, directions to the trail, trailhead coordinates, a trail map, an elevation profile, and a trail description. Many also include a note on nearby activities. Combined, the maps and information provide a clear method to assess each trail from the comfort of your favorite reading chair.

IN BRIEF

A "taste of the trail." Think of this section as a snapshot focused on the historical landmarks, beautiful vistas, and other sights you may encounter on the hike.

KEY AT-A-GLANCE INFORMATION

The information in the key at-a-glance boxes gives you a quick idea of the statistics and specifics of each hike.

LENGTH The length of the trail from start to finish (total distance traveled). There may be options to shorten or extend the hikes, but the mileage corresponds to the described hike. Consult the hike description to help decide how to customize the hike for your ability or time constraints.

CONFIGURATION A description of what the trail might look like from overhead. Trails can be loops, out-and-backs (trails on which one enters and leaves along the same path), figure eights, or a combination of shapes.

DIFFICULTY The degree of effort an "average" hiker should expect on a given hike. For simplicity, the trails are rated as "easy," "moderate," or "difficult."

SCENERY A short summary of the attractions offered by the hike and what to expect in terms of plant life, wildlife, natural wonders, and historic features.

EXPOSURE A quick check of how much sun you can expect on your shoulders during the hike.

TRAFFIC Indicates how busy the trail might be on an average day. Trail traffic, of course, varies from day to day and season to season. Weekend days typically see the most visitors. Other types of trail users you may encounter on the trail are also noted here.

TRAIL SURFACE Indicates whether the trail surface is paved, rocky, gravel, dirt, boardwalk, or a mixture of elements.

HIKING TIME The length of time it takes to hike the trail. A slow but steady hiker will average 2 to 3 miles an hour, depending on the terrain.

ACCESS A notation of any fees or permits that may be needed to access the trail or park at the trailhead.

MAPS Here you'll find a list of maps that show the topography of the trail, including Green Trails Maps and USGS topo maps.

FACILITIES What to expect in terms of restrooms and water at the trailhead or nearby.

DIRECTIONS

Used in conjunction with the overview map, the driving directions will help you locate each trailhead. Once at the trailhead, park only in designated areas.

GPS TRAILHEAD COORDINATES

The trailhead coordinates can be used in addition to the driving directions if you enter the coordinates into your GPS unit before you set out. See page 2 for more information on GPS coordinates.

DESCRIPTION

The trail description is the heart of each hike. Here, the authors provide a summary of the trail's essence and highlight any special traits the hike has to offer. The route is clearly outlined, including landmarks, side trips, and possible alternate routes along the way. Ultimately, the hike description will help you choose which hikes are best for you.

NEARBY ACTIVITIES

Look here for information on nearby activities or points of interest. This includes nearby parks, museums, restaurants, or even a brewpub where you can get a well-deserved beer after a long hike. Note that not every hike has a listing.

WEATHER

One of Atlanta's best-kept secrets is its weather. During the winter, warm days and cool evenings are the norm, although there are usually at least a couple of cold spells, rarely lasting more than two or three days. As the mercury slides up the thermometer in summer, average temperatures spend two months near the 90°F mark, which is when many hikers head for north Georgia, where temps can average 3°F to 5°F less. Extremes aside, summer and winter are full of mild days that provide excellent opportunities for hiking. For those who like to watch leaves change, flowers bloom, and birds migrate, spring and fall are a favorite time for a ramble.

Although the seasons provide a bounty of possible weather conditions, there are sometimes major weather variations within the region. When local forecasters talk about the "wedge of (cooler/warmer/drier) air," they are talking about a phenomenon created by the unique geography of the area. The Blue Ridge Mountains and the Atlantic Ocean create a weather system between them that frequently extends past the city to the border of Alabama. It is most noticeable when the air in Georgia is drier than the air in Alabama and a rain shower evaporates as it reaches the Alabama–Georgia border.

With all these variations in Atlanta weather, the word to remember is adaptability. If you want to continue hiking all year, it helps to have apparel for a range of conditions. Especially in winter and early spring, consider bringing an extra layer of clothing. Even on a warm spring or fall day, a trip to the mountains may require a light windbreaker. Adaptability, however, is not just a question of wearing sandals or snowshoes, hiking shorts or insulated pants—it's also an attitude. Being adaptable means thinking less about how the weather ought to be and thinking more about ways to find pleasure in a variety of conditions.

Average Temperature by Month

	Jan	Feb	Mar	Apr	May	Jun
High	52°	57°	65°	73°	80°	87°
Low	33°	37°	44°	50°	59°	67°
	Jul	Aug	Sep	Oct	Nov	Dec
High	89°	88°	82°	73°	63°	55°
Low	71°	70°	64°	53°	44°	36°

WATER

How much is enough? Well, one simple physiological fact should convince you to err on the side of excess when deciding how much water to pack: A hiker working hard in 90°F heat needs approximately ten quarts of fluid per day. That's 2.5 gallons—12 large water bottles or 16 small ones. In other words, pack along one or two bottles even for short hikes.

Some hikers and backpackers hit the trail prepared to purify water found along the route. This method, while less dangerous than drinking it untreated, comes with risks. Purifiers with ceramic filters are the safest. Many hikers pack along the slightly distasteful tetraglycine-hydroperiodide tablets to de-bug water (sold under the names Potable Aqua, Coghlan's, and others).

Probably the most common waterborne "bug" that hikers face is giardia, which may not hit until one to four weeks after ingestion. It will have you living in the bathroom, passing noxious rotten-egg gas, vomiting, and shivering with chills. Other parasites to worry about include E. coli and cryptosporidium, both of which are harder to kill than giardia.

For most people, the pleasures of hiking make carrying water a relatively minor price to pay to remain healthy. If you're tempted to drink "found water," do so only if you understand the risks involved. Better yet, hydrate before hiking, carry (and drink) six ounces of water for every mile you plan to hike, and hydrate after the hike.

CLOTHING

The most important thing to remember is that you want to be comfortable on the trail, and being comfortable means keeping yourself cool in summer and warm in winter. In warmer weather, you might try Under Armour, which offers summer wear T-shirts with incredible "wicking"; shorts are popular for their loose, comfortable fit. If you'll be in the grasslands or woodlands, consider opting for a pair of hiking pants; they'll help protect your legs from the ticks and snakes commonly found in these areas. You can find lightweight, quick-drying, UV-protective pants at many outdoors shops that will keep you suitably cool. Consider a pair that converts into shorts so that you can unzip them when you're done with the trail.

Hiking in cooler weather brings its own set of problems because, even though it might be cold out, after a little exertion, you'll find yourself sweating. Layering is a good solution, and an important part of keeping you comfortable. Wear an Under Armour winter T-shirt as a base (again, for the incredible wicking), and top it with a lightweight fleece or sweater. In winter, add an outer jacket. It's more than likely you'll find yourself taking off and putting on layers throughout the hike.

Year-round you'll want to be sure you have a good pair of hiking shoes. Day hikers are a great choice for most Atlanta-area trails. They come in both low-top and high-top, and are lightweight but have good tread and support. Tennis shoes are suitable for any of the paved trails, but are not ideal for the dirt paths. A hat is essential at any time of the year, and not only keeps the Georgia sun from burning your face, but also doubles as protection against insects and low-hanging limbs. Another useful item is a rain jacket that can be compressed small enough to be stuffed in your pack; if you're caught out in the rain, you'll be thankful for it.

THE TEN ESSENTIALS

One of the first rules of hiking is to be prepared for anything. The simplest way to be prepared is to carry the "Ten Essentials." In addition to carrying the items listed below, you need to know how to use them, especially navigation items. Always consider worst-case scenarios like getting lost, hiking back in the dark, breaking gear (for example, breaking a hip strap on your pack or finding a water filter got plugged), twisting an ankle, or encountering a brutal thunderstorm. The items listed below don't cost a lot of money, don't take up much room in a pack, and don't weigh much, but they might just save your life.

Water: durable bottles, and water treatment like iodine or a filter

Map: preferably a topo map and a trail map with a route description

Compass: a high-quality compass

First-aid kit: a good-quality kit including first-aid instructions

Knife: a multitool device with pliers is best

Light: flashlight or headlamp with extra bulbs and batteries

Fire: windproof matches or lighter and fire starter

Extra food: You should always have food in your pack when you've finished hiking.

Extra clothes: rain protection, warm layers, gloves, warm hat

Sun protection: sunglasses, lip balm, sunblock, sun hat

FIRST-AID KIT

A typical first-aid kit may contain more items than you might think necessary. These are just the basics. Prepackaged kits in waterproof bags (Atwater Carey and Adventure Medical make a variety of kits) are available. Even though there are quite a few items listed here, they pack down into a small space:

Ace bandages or Spenco joint wraps

Antibiotic ointment (Neosporin or the generic equivalent)

Aspirin or acetaminophen

Band-Aids

Benadryl or the generic equivalent diphenhydramine (in case of allergic reactions)

Butterfly-closure bandages

Epinephrine in a prefilled syringe (for people known to have severe allergic
   reactions to such things as bee stings)

Gauze (one roll)

Gauze compress pads (a half dozen 4 x 4-inch pads)

Hydrogen peroxide or iodine

Insect repellent

Matches or pocket lighter

Moleskin/Spenco 2ndSkin

Sunscreen

Whistle (it's more effective in signaling rescuers than your voice is)

HIKING WITH CHILDREN

No one is too young for a hike in the outdoors. Be mindful, though. Flat, short, and shaded trails are best with an infant. Toddlers who have not quite mastered walking can still tag along, riding on an adult's back in a child carrier. Use common sense to judge a child's capacity to hike a particular trail, and always expect that the child will tire quickly and need to be carried.

When packing for the hike, remember the child's needs in addition to your own. Make sure children are adequately clothed for the weather, have proper shoes, and are protected from the sun with sunscreen. Kids dehydrate quickly, so make sure you have plenty of fluid for everyone. To help you determine which trails are suitable for children, we list hikes suitable for children on page xvi.

GENERAL SAFETY

While many folks hit the trails full of enthusiasm and energy, eager to begin their adventures, others may find themselves more reserved about potential outdoor hazards. Although potentially dangerous situations can occur anywhere, your hike can be as safe and enjoyable as you hoped, as long as you use sound judgment and prepare yourself before hitting the trail. Here are a few tips to make your trip safer and easier:

- Hike with a buddy. Not only is there safety in numbers, but a buddy can help you if you twist an ankle on the trail or if you get lost, can assist in carrying lunch and water, and can be there to share in your discoveries. If you're hiking alone, be sure you've left your hiking itinerary with a friend or relative. Use common sense. Never enter the vehicle of someone you meet on the trail. It's best to bring a buddy not only to infrequently traveled or remote areas but also to urban areas.

- Stay hydrated. Georgia heat and humidity can sometimes be brutal, and a little exertion can quickly have you sweating. Don't wait until you feel thirsty; instead drink plenty of water throughout the hike, and at regular intervals.

- Always carry food and water whether you are planning to go overnight or not. Food will give you energy, help keep you warm, and sustain you in an emergency situation until help arrives. You never know if you will have a stream nearby when you become thirsty. Bring potable water or treat water before drinking it from a stream. Boil or filter all found water before drinking it.

- Stay on designated trails. Most hikers get lost when they leave the path. Even on the most clearly marked trails, there is usually a point where you have to stop and consider which direction to head. If you become disoriented, don't panic. As soon as you think you may be off-track, stop, assess your current direction, and then retrace your steps to the point where you went astray. Using your map, compass, and this book, and keeping in mind what you passed to that point, reorient yourself, and trust your judgment about how to continue. If you become absolutely unsure of where to go, return to your vehicle the way you came in. Should you become completely lost and have no idea how to return to the trailhead, stopping where you are on the trail and waiting for help is most often the best option for adults and always the best option for children.

- Be especially careful when crossing streams. Whether you are fording the stream or crossing on a log, make every step count. If you have any doubt about maintaining your balance on a foot log, go ahead and ford the stream instead. When fording a stream, use a trekking pole or stout stick for balance and face upstream as you cross. If a stream seems too deep to ford, turn back. Whatever is on the other side is not worth risking your life for.

- Be careful at overlooks. Although these areas may provide spectacular views, they are potentially hazardous. Stay back from the edge of outcrops and be absolutely sure of your footing; a misstep can mean a nasty and possibly fatal fall.

- Standing dead trees and storm-damaged living trees pose a real hazard to hikers and tent campers. These trees may have loose or broken limbs that could fall at any time. When choosing a spot to rest or selecting a backcountry campsite, look up.

- Know the symptoms of heat exhaustion. Sweating excessively, feeling faint or dizzy, getting clammy skin, vomiting, and becoming pale are all common symptoms. If symptoms arise, cool the person off by removing extra clothing, moving him or her to the shade, and offering water.

- Know the symptoms of hypothermia. Shivering and forgetfulness are the two most common indicators of this insidious killer. Hypothermia can occur at any elevation, even in the summer, especially when the hiker is wearing lightweight cotton clothing. If symptoms arise, get the victim shelter, hot liquids, and dry clothes or a dry sleeping bag.

- Take along your brain. A cool, calculating mind is the single most important equipment you'll ever want on the trail. Think before you act. Watch your step. Plan ahead. Avoiding accidents before they happen is the best way to ensure a rewarding and relaxing hike.

- Ask questions. Visitor center and park employees are there to help. It's a lot easier to get advice beforehand and avoid a mishap away from civilization when it's too late to amend an error. Use your head on the trail and be as kind to each area as you would if it were your own backyard.

ANIMAL AND PLANT HAZARDS
TICKS

Ticks are often found on brush and tall grass, where they wait to hitch a ride on a warm-blooded passerby. They become more common in the warm spring in the Atlanta area, and are a problem throughout the summer. Their numbers dwindle in the fall, but in Atlanta it is possible to get infected with a tick-borne disease any month of the year. Among the local varieties of ticks, the ones that transmit diseases are American dog ticks, the Lone Star tick, and the black-legged tick (deer tick). These ticks need to attach for several hours before they can transmit disease.

Deer ticks are the primary carrier of Lyme disease, and others carry Rocky Mountain spotted fever and tick-related monocytic ehrlichiosis. Insect repellent containing Deet is known to be an effective deterrent. Most importantly, though, be sure to visually check yourself at the end of the hike. If it's prime tick season, you may want to perform a quick check every hour or so. During your post-hike shower, take a moment to do a more complete body check. For ticks that are already embedded, it is best to remove them with tweezers.

SNAKES

Spend some time hiking in Atlanta and you may be surprised by the variety of snakes in the area. Most encounters will be with nonvenomous specimens, like the Eastern garter and king snake. Atlanta does have its share of venomous snakes, but the only ones we have seen on the trail are the diamondback rattlesnake and the copperhead. Coral

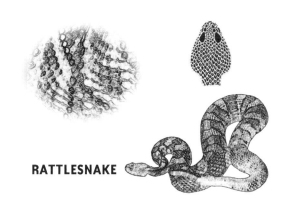

RATTLESNAKE

snakes are surprisingly common in lakes, though sightings of this smaller rattler are rare. You might spend a few minutes studying snakes before heading into the woods, but a good rule of thumb is to give whatever animal you encounter a wide berth and leave it alone.

POISON IVY/POISON OAK/ POISON SUMAC

Recognizing poison ivy, poison oak, and poison sumac and avoiding contact with them is the most effective way to prevent the painful, itchy rashes associated with these plants. In the Southeast, poison ivy ranges from a thick, tree-hugging vine to a shaded ground cover, three leaflets to a leaf; poison oak occurs as either a vine or shrub, also with three leaflets; and poison sumac flourishes in swampland, with each leaf having 7 to 13 leaflets. Urushiol, the oil in the sap of these plants, is responsible

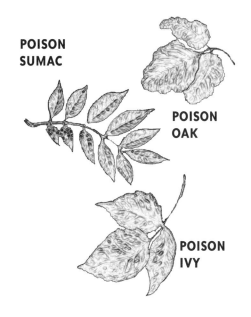

POISON SUMAC

POISON OAK

POISON IVY

for the rash. Usually within 12 to 14 hours of one's exposure (but sometimes much later), raised lines and/or blisters will appear, accompanied by a terrible itch. Refrain from scratching because bacteria under fingernails can cause infection and you will spread the rash to other parts of your body. Wash and dry the rash thoroughly, applying a calamine lotion or other product to help dry the rash out. If itching or blistering is severe, seek medical attention. Remember that oil-contaminated clothes, pets, or hiking gear can easily cause an irritating rash on you or someone else, so wash not only any exposed parts of your body but also clothes, gear, and pets.

MOSQUITOES

Although it's not common, people can become infected with the West Nile virus by being bitten by an infected mosquito. Culex mosquitoes, the primary variety that transmits West Nile virus to humans, thrive in urban rather than natural areas. They lay their eggs in stagnant water and can breed in any standing water that remains for more than five days. Most people infected with West Nile virus have no symptoms of illness, but some may become ill, usually 3 to 15 days after being bitten.

In Atlanta the summer months bring mosquitoes, and with them the highest risk periods for West Nile virus. Mosquitoes are especially prevalent on trails with tall grasses, in marshy or swampy areas, and at dusk and dawn. Any time you expect mosquitoes to be buzzing around, you may want to wear protective clothing, such as long sleeves, long pants, and socks. Loose-fitting, light-colored clothing is best. Spray clothing with insect repellent. The Centers for Disease Control and Prevention (CDC) acknowledges that repellents containing the active ingredients Deet or Picardin offer the best protection; they also suggest oil of lemon eucalyptus is an effective plant-based repellent. Remember to follow the instructions on the repellent and to take extra care with children. Within the past few years, insect-repellent clothing has come on the market and is available at most outdoor retailer shops.

TIPS FOR ENJOYING ATLANTA

If you plan on hiking in one of the state parks or the national forests, visit their Web sites for information to help you get oriented to your destination's roads, features, and attractions . General and detailed maps of the specific wilderness areas are often available online or at the state park's office. (See "Contact Information" at the end of this book). In addition, the following tips will make your visit enjoyable and more rewarding:

- **Be sure you get out of your car and onto a trail. Auto touring allows a cursory and largely visual overview of the area. On the trail you can use your ears and nose as well. Even if you don't use the trails recommended in this guidebook, any trail is better than no trail at all. Summer days in Atlanta can be hot. If there's a nice day you just don't want to miss out on because of** the heat, go early in the morning. If you're on the trail at dawn, you can find temperatures 10ºF to 20ºF degrees lower than they'll be later in the day, and there's no better way to start your day than by listening to the cheerful singing of birds as you hike.

- Take your time along the trails. Pace yourself. Atlanta is filled with wonders both big, such as Amicalola Falls, and small, such as an antebellum shed now used as a garage. Don't rush past a tiny lizard to get to that overlook. Stop and smell the wildflowers. Peer into a clear creek for minnows. Don't miss the trees for the forest. Shorter hikes allow you to stop and linger more than long hikes do. Something about staring at the front end of a 10-mile trek naturally pushes you to speed up. That said, take close notice of the elevation maps that accompany each hike. If you see many ups and downs over large altitude changes, you'll obviously need more time. Inevitably, you'll finish some of the hikes long before (or after) the estimated hiking time. Nevertheless, leave yourself plenty of time for those moments when you simply feel like stopping and taking it all in.

- We can't always schedule time off when we want it, but try to hike during the week and avoid the traditional holidays, if possible. Trails that are packed in the spring and fall are often clear during the hotter or colder months. If you are hiking on a busy day, go early in the morning; it'll enhance your chances of seeing wildlife. The trails really clear out during rainy times; however, don't hike during a thunderstorm. After a storm, hike a trail with a waterfall to enjoy the falls at full volume.

- Investigate different areas around Atlanta. The scenery you'll find hiking through meadows and grasslands is pleasantly different from that in the riparian forest along a fork of the Chattahoochee River, and different still from lakeside water views. Sample a few hikes in each area to see what it has to offer and what most appeals to you.

- Hike during different seasons. Trails change dramatically from spring to winter, sometimes transforming themselves into something you might not even recognize. If you found a trail you particularly liked—or didn't—try it in a different season.

- Hike a loop trail backward. Hiking a trail in both directions gives new views of an old trail. Watch for scenic views that may not have been obvious when you hiked the path as outlined in the book, but be aware that the hike can be harder.

TOPO MAPS

The maps in this book have been produced with great care and, used with the hiking directions, will direct you to the trail and help you stay on course. However, you will find superior detail and valuable information in the United States Geological Survey's 7.5-minute series topographic maps. Topo maps are available online in many locations. A well-known free service is at **www.terraserver.microsoft.com** and another free service, with fast click-and-drag browsing, is at **www.topofinder .com.** You can view and print topos of the entire United States from these Web sites, and view aerial photographs of the same area at **terraserver.com.** Several online services, such as **www.trails.com,** charge annual fees for additional features such as shaded-relief, which makes the altitude changes stand out more. If you expect to print out many topo maps each year, it might be worth paying for shaded-relief topo maps. The downside to USGS topos is that most of them are outdated, having been created 20 to 30 years ago. But they still provide excellent topographic detail.

Digital topographic map programs, such as Delorme's TopoUSA, enable you to review topo maps of the entire United States on your PC. Gathered while hiking with a GPS unit, the GPS data can also be downloaded into the software and used to plot your own hikes.

If you're new to hiking, you might be wondering, "What's a topographic map?" In short, a topo indicates not only linear distance but elevation as well, using contour lines. Contour lines extend across the map like dozens of intricate spiderwebs. Each line represents a particular elevation, and at the base of each topo, a contour's interval designation is given. If the contour interval is 20 feet, then the distance between each contour line is 20 feet. Follow five contour lines up on the same map, and the elevation has increased by 100 feet.

Let's assume that the 7.5-minute series topo reads "Contour Interval 40 feet," that the short trail we'll be hiking is two inches long on the map, and that the trail crosses five contour lines from beginning to end. What do we know? Well, because the linear scale of this series is 2,000 feet to the inch (roughly 2.75 inches:1 mile), we know our trail is approximately 0.8 miles long (2 inches:2,000 feet). But we also know we'll be climbing or descending 200 vertical feet (five contour lines, at 40 feet each) over that distance. And the elevation designations written on occasional contour lines will tell us if we're heading up or down.

In addition to the outdoor shops listed in the Appendix, major universities and some public libraries also have topos; you might try photocopying the ones you need to avoid the cost of buying them. But if you want your own and can't find them locally, visit the United States Geological Survey Web site at **topomaps.usgs.gov.**

BACKCOUNTRY/PRIMITIVE CAMPING ADVICE

Backcountry or primitive camping is available in the Chattahoochee National Forest, and in many state parks and wildlife management areas. You should always practice low-impact camping. Adhere to the adages "Pack it in, pack it out," and "Take only pictures, leave only footprints." "Leave no trace" ethics make hiking (and camping) more fun for others . Some backcountry areas are also public hunting areas, so be sure to ask for hunting season times and wear hunter's orange during these periods.

Solid human waste should be buried in a hole at least three inches deep and at least 200 feet away from trails and water sources; a trowel is basic backpacking equipment.

Rules on open fires vary depending on where you go, so you'll want to check before your visit; when collecting firewood, many places ask you to collect downed wood instead of chopping branches. In addition, Georgia State Parks allow fires only in fire rings, fireplaces, and campsite grills. Burn bans, especially during drought periods, can restrict fires—including those at campsite grills. Be sure to double-check before your trip because state parks may or may not be affected by a countywide burn ban.

A fishing license is required if you plan on fishing. You can get one from many outdoor retailers, sports stores, and bait and tackle shops; online; or over the phone. Visit the Georgia Wildlife Resources Web site **georgiawildlife.dnr .state.ga.us** for information on regulations, fees, permits, and purchase.

Following the above guidelines will help you ensure a pleasant, safe, and low-impact interaction between you and the rest of nature. These suggestions are intended to enhance your experience. Regulations can change over time; contact the appropriate park office to confirm the status of any regulations before you enter the backcountry.

TRAIL ETIQUETTE

Whether you're on a city, county, state, or national park trail, always remember that great care and resources (from nature and from your tax dollars) have gone into creating these trails. Treat the trail, wildlife, and fellow hikers with respect.

- **Hike on open trails only. Respect trail and road closures (ask if not sure), avoid trespassing on private land, and obtain all permits and authorization as required. Also, leave gates as you found them or as marked.**

- **Leave only footprints. Be sensitive to the ground beneath you. This also means staying on the existing trail and not blazing new trails. Be sure to pack out what you pack in. No one likes to see the trash someone else has left behind.**

- **Never spook animals. An unannounced approach, a sudden movement, or a loud noise startles most animals. A surprised animal can be dangerous to you, to others, and to itself. Give wildlife plenty of space.**

- **Plan ahead. Know your equipment, your ability, and the area in which you are hiking—and prepare accordingly. Be self-sufficient at all times; carry necessary supplies for changes in weather or other conditions. A well-executed trip is satisfying to you and to others.**

- **Be courteous to other hikers, bikers, equestrians, and others you encounter on the trails.**

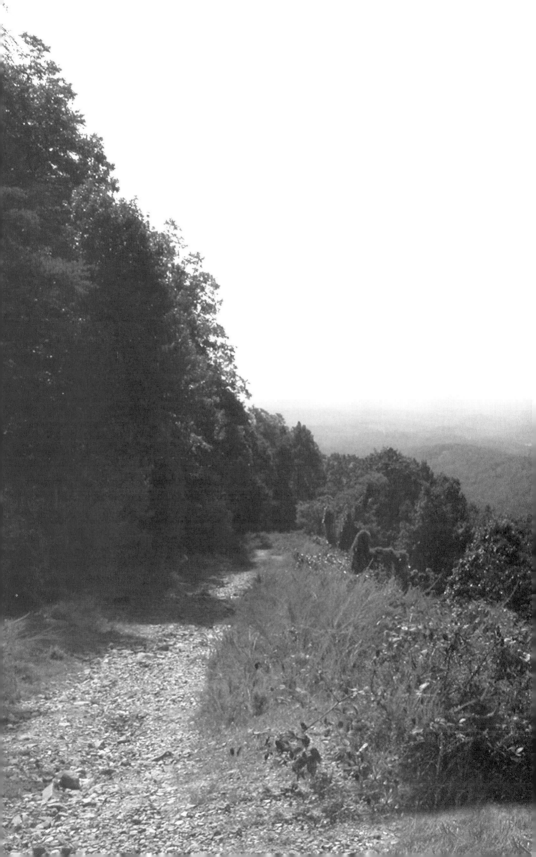

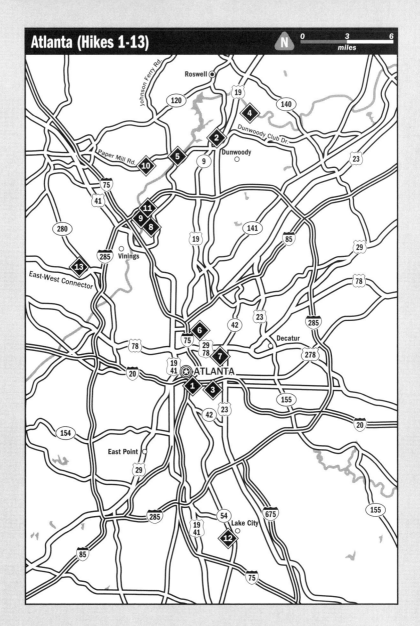

ATLANTA

01 ATLANTA RAMBLE

KEY AT-A-GLANCE INFORMATION

LENGTH: 5.4 miles
CONFIGURATION: Loop
DIFFICULTY: Easy
SCENERY: Urban scenes, including high-rise buildings
EXPOSURE: Full sun
TRAFFIC: Heavy
TRAIL SURFACE: Concrete sidewalks
HIKING TIME: 5 hours
ACCESS: Open year-round
MAPS: Atlanta Convention and Visitors Bureau; Atlanta Chamber of Commerce; USGS Southwest Atlanta, Northwest Atlanta
FACILITIES: All necessary facilities found throughout
SPECIAL COMMENTS: Underground Atlanta has a number of excellent restaurants.

IN BRIEF

From Ted Turner Field, this hike visits the capital dome, Underground Atlanta, Georgia Dome, Phillips Arena, CNN Center, Centennial Park, the Georgia Aquarium, and the World of Coca-Cola.

DESCRIPTION

This hike begins in the parking lot opposite Turner Field, at the site of the original Atlanta–Fulton County Stadium. From the parking lot is a great view of downtown Atlanta and the Olympic flame. Turner Field was built to house the Olympics and then converted into a baseball field to replace the aging Fulton County Stadium. A plaque commemorates the most historic moment that occurred at the original structure, Henry (Hank) Aaron's 715th home run, which he hit on April 6, 1974, breaking Babe Ruth's long-standing record.

Turn around, cross Georgia Avenue, and enter Turner Field at the black iron gates. Purchase tickets for the tour in the box office, and view the Braves Hall of Fame museum before the tour. In addition to a World Series trophy, they have a railroad car the Braves used in the 1950s and a display on the various fields in which the Braves have played. The tour visits the Braves dugout and bullpen, and takes you next to the ball field and

UTM Trailhead Coordinates

UTM Zone (NAD27) 16S

Easting   0741854

Northing   3736068

Directions

Take Interstate 75/Interstate 85 South to Exit 246 (Fulton Street). At the end of the ramp, turn left and travel 0.2 miles. Turn right on Hank Aaron Drive (also known as Capitol Avenue). At Georgia Avenue turn right again and enter the Green lot on the right.

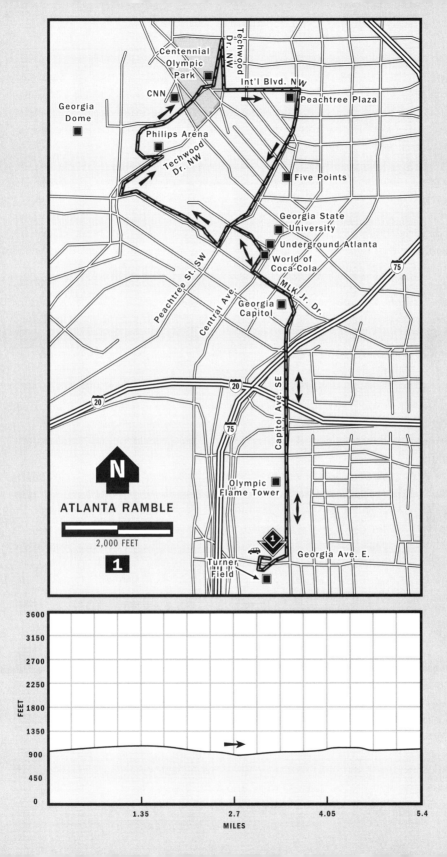

then into the locker room. Off-season hours are Monday through Saturday from 10 a.m. to 2 p.m. Beginning April 1, tours are offered Monday through Saturday from 9 a.m. to 3 p.m. and Sunday from 1 p.m. to 3 p.m. On game days, tours are offered from 9 a.m. to noon. Tours start on the hour and last about an hour.

When exiting Turner Field, turn right on Georgia Avenue, then turn left on Henry Aaron Drive, crossing under the Olympic rings and passing the flame on your left. At 0.9 miles the Georgia State Capitol is on the left. Inside the building, which is open from 8 a.m. to 5 p.m. Monday through Friday, is a large number of displays about the cultural and natural history of Georgia, including Georgia's role in the civil rights movement. On the grounds are statues of some fairly well-known Georgia politicians, including Jimmy Carter, Richard B. Russell, and John B. Gordon, among others. After looping around the grounds, return to MLK Drive, cross the street, and turn left. On the corner of MLK and Washington Street, notice the statue to the working dogs whose heroism saved many lives during the terrorist attacks on the World Trade Center in New York City. After crossing Central Avenue, you will see the old World of Coca-Cola building on the right, which marks the start of Underground Atlanta.

As you leave the area, look across an open area for a mural of whales. Below that is the 1869 Atlanta Depot, now an upscale restaurant. When this freight depot was completed, it was the tallest building in Atlanta, but a 1935 fire destroyed the second floor. Turn left just before the depot and enter Underground Atlanta.

A potpourri of shops, restaurants, and nightclubs, the three-level Underground Atlanta is a vast underground city within a city. Directly in front of you is an information kiosk and many restaurants. Underground Atlanta was created at the start of the 20th century, when the population of Atlanta had soared to 200,000 people. Crossing the tracks through downtown had become a major traffic snarl, so the government added an iron bridge to speed up traffic. In 1929 the iron bridge was converted into a concrete viaduct, and businesses moved their storefronts to the second story of the buildings.

At the end of the food court, turn left and take the escalator to Kenny's Alley. Turn left again and stroll down Upper Alabama Street to Peachtree Street just south of Five Points. Turn left on Peachtree and right on MLK Drive, and walk 0.4 miles to Centennial Olympic Park Drive. Directly in front of you is the white-roofed, red-sided Georgia Dome, home of the Atlanta Falcons. Turn right on Centennial Drive and continue past the MARTA station until you are standing directly in front of Phillips Arena. This new site is the home to both the Atlanta Hawks and the Atlanta Thrashers and is a popular concert venue. Note the word "Atlanta" spelled in white letters in the front of the building. Turn around and walk back to the first road on the right, and turn right.

At the end of this road is one of the three massive buildings that comprise the Georgia World Congress Center (GWCC). Built on the site of the old Atlanta

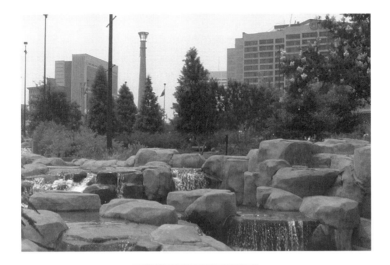

Centennial Olympic Park

roundhouse, the Congress Center is home to hundreds of industry shows a year. It was this area that was heavily damaged in the 2008 Atlanta Tornado. Turn right and continue down International Boulevard, passing the CNN Center and Omni Hotel on the right and the Atlanta Chamber of Commerce on the left.

You are now in the center of Atlanta's Centennial Olympic Park. Designed by EDAW and built by Beers-Russell, the park features the Fountain of Rings, the Great Lawn, a water garden, and five unique "quilt plazas" telling the story of the Atlanta Olympics; the Quilt of Remembrance was designed to tell the story of the bombing that killed 2 people and injured 118 more in the park. After viewing the Fountain of Rings on the right, turn left and walk to the reflecting pool. With the pool on your immediate left, there is a trail almost directly in front of you. This leads to the Water Gardens, our favorite part of the park. Follow the path 0.1 mile to reach the Georgia Agricultural Plaza on Baker Street. The Georgia Aquarium, the world's largest aquarium, opened in November 2005. Within the aquarium are five areas, including Cold Water Quest, Georgia Explorer, Ocean Voyager, River Scout, and Tropical Diver.

The World of Coca-Cola, next to the aquarium, is a multimedia presentation designed to both educate and fascinate visitors. Exhibiting early print ads, modern TV commercials, and everything in between, the displays take visitors through the development of Coca-Cola's image and products. Turn right on Baker, right again on Centennial Olympic Park Drive, and then left on Andrew Young International Boulevard. On the left are the Gift Mart and the Merchandise Mart. On the right is the impressive 72-story Westin Peachtree Plaza, a fixture of the Atlanta skyline and home of the most exciting elevator ride in the southeastern United

States. The ride climbs the outside of the building, affording a complete view of the city. At the top, the Sundial restaurant and lounge makes a complete revolution every hour.

Turn right (south) on Peachtree Street, Atlanta's main boulevard. When the Fulton County Library comes into view just south of Carnegie Way, you are entering the oldest area of Atlanta, known as the Fairlie-Poplar district. It was here that the first residential homes were constructed, to be replaced by commercial structures after the Civil War. Today the district is an amalgam of old and new buildings blending together almost seamlessly. Continuing south on Peachtree, you'll see Woodruff Park on the left. Watch for the Coca-Cola Spectacular, followed by Five Points, created by the intersection of Peachtree, Marietta, and Decatur Streets and Edgewood Avenue. Continue south on Peachtree two more blocks and turn left into Underground Atlanta. From this point, retrace your steps to Turner Field.

NEARBY ATTRACTIONS

The APEX Museum on Auburn Avenue looks at the history of African Americans in the city of Atlanta. Fittingly situated on Auburn Avenue, the economic and cultural center for African Americans when Atlanta was segregated, the museum explores the economic and cultural rise of the Sweet Auburn district. Turn left two blocks after Carnegie Way on Auburn Avenue. The museum is two blocks down on your right and is open in February and from June through August only, Tuesday through Saturday, from 10 a.m. to 5 p.m., and Sunday, from 1 p.m. to 5 p.m.

BIG TREES PRESERVE TRAIL

IN BRIEF

Big Trees has multiple loops and straight-line trails that can be combined for a wide variety of hikes. A 300-foot climb on the Backcountry Loop is so well done it seems effortless.

DESCRIPTION

The John Ripley Forbes Big Trees Forest Preserve was created and is managed by the Southeast Land Preservation Trust in partnership with both Fulton County and the State of Georgia, which technically own the land. At 30 acres, it is one of the largest undeveloped tracts in the city of Sandy Springs, north of Atlanta. It is named in honor of John Ripley Forbes, a naturalist who worked extensively with local governments nationwide to preserve land. Mr. Forbes's legacy in Atlanta includes both Fernbank Museum and the Chattahoochee Nature Center.

From the trailhead, the paved path begins an easy descent into the Powers Branch watershed. Immediately visible to the right is the pre-1902 roadbed of Roswell Road, a major Atlanta-area road that permitted Roswell-area mills access to the railhead in Atlanta and served every town north of the Chattahoochee.

Directions →

Take GA 400 north to Exit 6, Northridge Road. Circle around and turn right at the end of the exit ramp. In 0.4 miles turn left on GA 9, known locally as Roswell Road. Continue south 1.4 miles to the North Fulton Annex, just past Morgan Falls Dam Road on the right. Turn left into the second (south) parking lot and look for the trailhead directly in front of you on the right.

KEY AT-A-GLANCE INFORMATION

LENGTH: 1.2 miles

CONFIGURATION: Loop

DIFFICULTY: Easy

SCENERY: Streamside and watershed views of Powers Branch

EXPOSURE: Mostly shaded

TRAFFIC: Moderate

TRAIL SURFACE: Packed dirt

HIKING TIME: 45 minutes

ACCESS: Open year-round, dawn–dusk

MAPS: Available at stand at trailhead. Look for a stapled, multi-page handout—the map is on the last page; USGS Chamblee.

FACILITIES: None

SPECIAL COMMENTS: Big Trees Trail parking can be crowded because it is also the parking lot for the North Fulton Annex. Dogs must be leashed at all times and cleaned up after; this is strictly enforced.

UTM Trailhead Coordinates

UTM Zone (NAD27) 16S

Easting 0743664

Northing 3761152

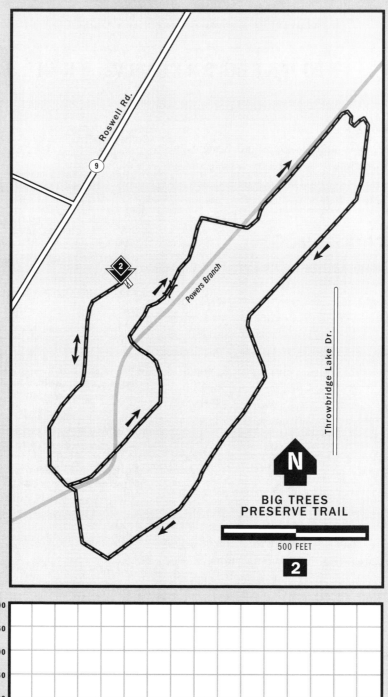

Roswell Rd.

9

2

Powers Branch

Throwbridge Lake Dr.

N

BIG TREES
PRESERVE TRAIL

500 FEET

2

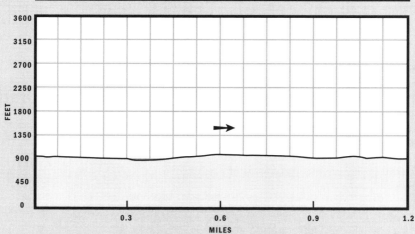

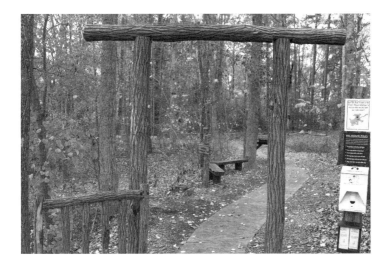

Big Trees Preserve Trail entrance

The Big Trees Loop splits at a marked intersection right up ahead. Continue straight on the split-rail fence–lined, chip-covered path as the paved trail bears left. As it descends, Big Trees Loop almost imperceptibly joins the old roadbed.

Bear right on Powers Branch Trail at 0.1 mile as Big Trees Loop Trail continues around to the left. As you descend to the creek, Beech Hollow Trail heads right, quickly falling to a loop around a massive American beech. At the bottom is a scenic side view of the creek near the culvert that carries the stream under the present-day Roswell Road. There are tree-stump seats, if you want to spend a few minutes in quiet reflection. As you return to Powers Branch Trail, turn right and descend to a 90-degree left-hand turn as the pathway joins Powers Branch. Continue straight when the Backcountry Connector heads right a few steps after the turn.

Over the next 0.2 miles, the trail climbs about 100 feet on an easy hike into the Powers Branch Watershed. The path twice crosses the stream: once on a wooden bridge, then on an interesting "rock hop"—a planned, raised rock path through the water. The stream runs through a concealed culvert underneath a large rock in the center. The kids will love this!

Just over 0.5 miles into the hike, the boulders get larger, but even an untrained eye can tell that the formation is not natural. On the left as you enter the area is an old road grade that disappears into the modern embankment of the North Fulton Annex. A small cascade in the river makes a pretty photograph, but the telltale drill hole gives away the secret—the falls are man-made. Just past the falls, Powers Branch Trail ends as Spring Hollow Trail turns right, crosses an unrailed bridge over the creek, and rises to the Backcountry Connector. Make a hard left at the end of the brief Spring Hollow Trail.

The Backcountry Connector continues to climb, paralleling the creek. As apartments come into view straight ahead, look down to the left. The creek is now 60 feet below the footpath. A few steps later the trail begins an easy double switch to climb to its highest point, just a few feet after the second switchback. From this point, the treadway begins an easy descent through a second-growth hardwood forest composed of white and post oak and American beech interspersed with native azalea.

As the hike approaches 1 mile, the footpath begins an easy curve to the right. At the end of the curve, the path runs adjacent to the grade of the Bull Sluice Railroad, built in 1902 to move material to the site of Morgan Falls Dam, one of the earliest hydroelectric projects in the state. After work on the dam was completed, the railbed was abandoned. At 1 mile a path to the left crosses a bridge and makes a switchback ascent to a patio adjacent to a Ford dealership. A small portion of this path actually runs on the level grade of the old railroad bed.

Just past this bridge is the left turn onto the short Backwoods Connector Trail. Cross a wooden bridge, turn to the left on Powers Branch Trail, and follow the path around to the right to return to the trailhead.

NEARBY ATTRACTIONS

Heritage Sandy Springs is an interpreted farmhouse and museum and the site of the five freshwater springs for which the city is named. The park, on Sandy Springs Circle just off Hammond Drive, is open daily from dawn to dusk.

GRANT PARK LOOP
(includes Zoo Atlanta)

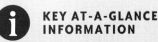

IN BRIEF

Grant Park Loop visits the 1880s-era green space that was the centerpiece of a development of wealthy homes. The park also houses Zoo Atlanta, which features animals living in near-native habitats.

DESCRIPTION

Each year, more than 2 million people visit Grant Park to see the world-class Zoo Atlanta, view a three-dimensional re-creation of the Civil War's Battle of Atlanta, see downtown from a Civil War fort, or just relax in the green space created by Lemuel Grant, for whom the park is named. Grant, who moved to Georgia from Maine in the late 1830s, was one of Atlanta's first citizens. He designed a series of defenses around the city that helped the Confederate army defend the city against a Union onslaught. After the Civil War, Grant played a key role in Atlanta's revitalization. He began organizing the park in 1881 and donated it to the city of Atlanta in 1883.

Grant Park has always been open to both blacks and whites, an unusual occurrence in the segregated South. Even the zoo was integrated—sort of. The Atlanta attraction regularly had "black-only" days. In 1921 Atlanta added the Cyclorama, a building to house the "Battle of Atlanta" painting. It also moved the Civil War locomotive *The Texas*, which had sat exposed in Grant Park, inside the building.

Directions

Take I-20 East to Exit 59A (Boulevard). At the end of the ramp, turn right and travel 0.4 miles to the parking lot on the right. If the parking lot is full, continue south on Boulevard to Atlanta Avenue; turn right, right again on Cherokee Street, and right into a second parking lot.

KEY AT-A-GLANCE INFORMATION

LENGTH: 3.1 miles

CONFIGURATION: Loop

DIFFICULTY: Easy

SCENERY: Well-kept, historic park with huge trees in a generally upscale downtown area

EXPOSURE: Partial shade to full sun

TRAFFIC: Heavy, especially in Zoo Atlanta

TRAIL SURFACE: Almost entirely paved

HIKING TIME: 3.5 hours

ACCESS: Open year-round

MAPS: Available at Zoo Atlanta; USGS Southeast Atlanta

FACILITIES: Restrooms, playgrounds, Civil War museum and Cyclorama; Zoo Atlanta

SPECIAL COMMENTS: This is a great family hike, featuring the zoo, playgrounds, and fast food.

UTM Trailhead Coordinates

UTM Zone (NAD27) 16S

Easting   0743764

Northing   3735747

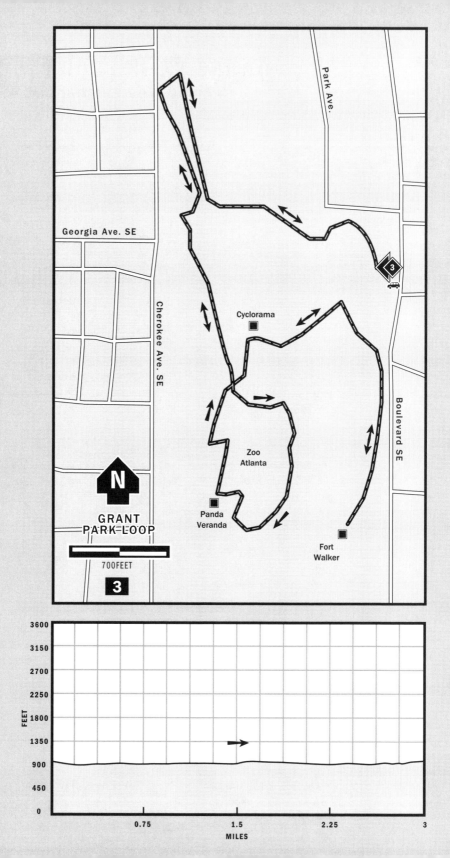

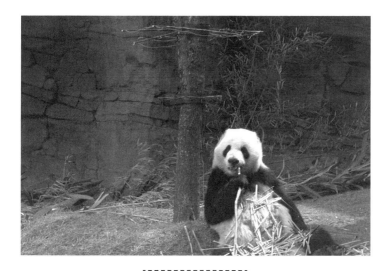

Panda at Zoo Atlanta

On a paved road across from the first lane of parking (the lane nearest the entrance), walk through four white posts underneath the spreading crowns of a group of old-growth post oaks. As the paved road begins an easy curve to the left, a side road leaves to the right. The road then curves back to the right as it heads toward a hill with a gazebo on top. Continue to bear right as the road splits in front of the gazebo, and you will reach a five-road intersection. Bear left on a road that descends then curves right. At 0.3 miles turn right. A few steps down this paved road is a small playground up on the right. As the road begins to rise, turn right on a paved road; immediately on the left is the massive stone fountain and a park entrance that was added in the early 1900s. Circle the structure, which is being restored by the Grant Park Conservancy, then make the first left and climb a short way to street level. Two roads enter Grant Park at 45-degree angles from Cherokee Avenue, which forms the eastern boundary of the park. This is a popular place to take a picture, but plan to get there later in the day and shoot from the far side of street. Continue to circle to the left, descending on the other side of the entrance.

At the end of the road, turn right at the T-intersection and climb to Cherokee Avenue for more views of both Grant Park and the surrounding neighborhood. The area is being rejuvenated thanks to low-interest loans from the city. Turn left and walk on the sidewalk, making the next left to head back into the park. As this road descends, it curves right, crossing a culvert on a concrete bridge. Just past the bridge is Constitution Spring, which was once one of five mineral springs within the park. A stone bridge sits in a tree-lined open field on the left of the road at 0.9 miles.

The road curves around to the left, coming out at the entrance to Zoo Atlanta. This nationally recognized zoo allows species to roam freely in specially designed areas intended to mimic the animal's natural habitat. Back in 1984, Atlantans discovered that the Metropolitan Zoo had been named one of the ten worst in the country. Some spoke of closing the zoo and returning Willie B., a silverback gorilla at the center of the controversy, to his home in Cameroon. Rather than give up, Atlanta hired a new director for the attraction, Terry Maples, who began the arduous task of completely rebuilding the zoo.

Stunning pink flamingos greet visitors just inside the entrance. Close by are elephants, the critically endangered black rhino, and a lion, then it's off to the Ford African Rain Forest. Willie B. died in 2000, but his offspring carry on the strong tradition of the rain forest in Atlanta, where multiple viewing sites allow glimpses into the lives of these stoic creatures. At the end of the rain forest, there are other animals and reptiles, but follow the path on the left just past a food kiosk to the panda exhibit for a one-of-a-kind treat.

Considered the symbol of peace in its homeland of China, the giant panda is a black-and-white fur-bearing mammal with markings similar to those of the raccoon, but DNA testing has proven it is in the bear family. Lun-Lun and Yang-Yang arrived at Zoo Atlanta in November 1999 for a ten-year stay and immediately became stars in the animal-oriented attraction. The endangered pandas occasionally play together, but mostly they eat bamboo in separate sections of their environment. A line forms quickly at this exhibit, so plan a 20- to 30-minute wait.

As you leave, the Panda Veranda is on the left, complete with picnic tables and a McDonald's. If you don't need a break, continue straight ahead to view the zoo's two Sumatran tigers. One of a handful of zoos with a captive breeding program, Zoo Atlanta is active in the fight to save this nearly extinct species. Fewer that 400 Sumatran tigers are known to exist in the wild or in captivity. As you exit the tiger exhibit, follow the road that bears left toward the Ford Pavilion, then follow the path to the right and turn right into the Kids Zone. Immediately after the turn is a marked railroad crossing for a train that young children can ride. Kids can get close to animals in the petting zoo and see kangaroos, but for our favorite exhibit, turn left at Base Camp Discovery and follow the path around to the left. Here, tortoises take their time exploring the habitat created by the zoo. These mammoth prehistoric beasts are fun to watch as they eat, sleep, or walk.

As you leave the Kids Zone, turn right; the exit is almost directly in front of you. After passing through the booths, on the left is the Cyclorama. Built in 1921, it houses a three-dimensional painting in the round, "The Battle of Atlanta," and a Civil War museum featuring *The Texas,* one of the locomotives involved in the Great Locomotive Chase.

After viewing the museum and the painting, exit and turn right. Turn right again on the first concrete path to wind back to the parking lot. Once in the parking lot, turn right and walk to the southern end of the lot. Follow the road around to the left and turn right on the paved path at the end of the second lane of parking. This path winds to Fort Walker, an earthen outpost along the defenses constructed by Grant. It is one of the few remaining intact Civil War sites in the Atlanta metropolitan area. From the top of the hill there is a good view of the downtown skyline. Return to the parking lot using the same path you followed to Fort Walker.

ISLAND FORD TRAIL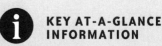

IN BRIEF

This hike explores the floodplain and watershed of the Chattahoochee River in the vicinity of Island Ford, one of the first commonly used fords of the river.

DESCRIPTION

Settlers normally had two options for crossing the Chattahoochee River. They could use one of the many ferries, which cost money, or one of the free fords, where animals, carts, and people made their way across a high, relatively flat area in the river. Fording the river could be a dangerous proposition. Fast-flowing, high water could easily drag a cart or person downriver. Eventually, a ferry did cross the river here.

When visiting the river today, it is next to impossible to find the actual location of the ford—the continuous flow requirement of Buford Dam keeps the water high enough to cover most of the rocky ledge the settlers used. When Jimmy Carter signed the act creating the Chattahoochee River National Recreation Area in 1978, the massive log home of Samuel Hewlett was designated park headquarters.

After parking your car, walk to the parking lot on the left as you face Hewlett's home. In the center of the lot, at a brown-roofed

KEY AT-A-GLANCE INFORMATION

LENGTH: 3.1 miles

CONFIGURATION: Loop

DIFFICULTY: Easy, with a couple of moderate climbs into the Chattahoochee River watershed

SCENERY: Riverbank views along the Chattahoochee

EXPOSURE: Mostly shaded, except in the area of a massive pine blowdown near the parking area

TRAFFIC: Moderate

TRAIL SURFACE: Compact soil

HIKING TIME: 1.5 hours

ACCESS: Open year-round, dawn–dusk; headquarters building open all year 9 a.m.–5 p.m.

MAPS: Map available in visitor center; USGS Chamblee

FACILITIES: Restrooms, ball field, some picnic tables, group pavilion

SPECIAL COMMENTS: Headquarters for the Chattahoochee River National Recreation Area (CRNRA) are located in the former home of Samuel Hewlett, who served on the Supreme Court of Georgia.

Directions

Take GA 400 north to Exit 6, Northridge Road. At the end of the ramp, get in the right-hand left-turn lane. Cross over GA 400 and make an immediate right at 0.1 mile, on Dunwoody Place. Merge left as the road becomes a single lane. At 0.5 miles turn right on Roberts Drive, which crosses back over GA 400. Turn right at the signed entrance to Island Ford. Proceed along the winding drive 1.2 miles to a parking lot at the end of the road.

UTM Trailhead Coordinates

UTM Zone (NAD27) 16S

Easting 0747036

Northing 3763769

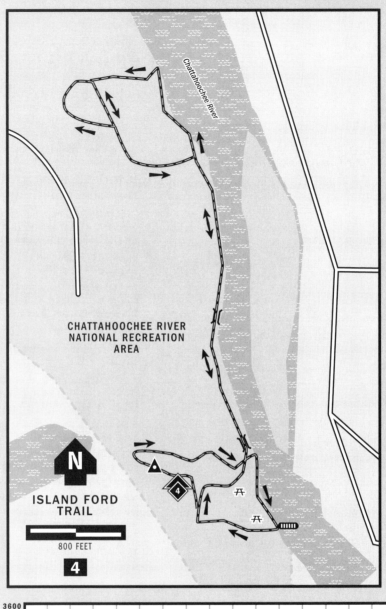

CHATTAHOOCHEE RIVER
NATIONAL RECREATION
AREA

Chattahoochee River

N

**ISLAND FORD
TRAIL**

800 FEET

4

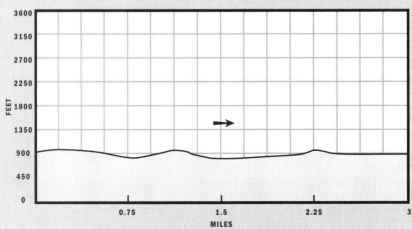

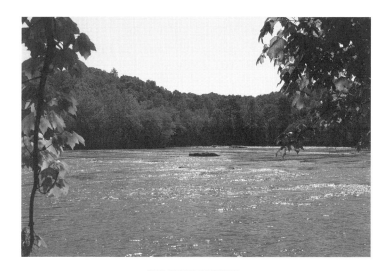

Island Ford Trail

information kiosk, is one of the entrances to the Island Ford Trail system. The trail initially falls to a small creek through a mostly pine forest with a variety of oak. Avoid the side trail you'll see on the right almost immediately after the start. At 0.2 miles the trail crosses Island Ford Road then comes to a small pond. Turn right to reach a wooden overlook a few steps away. After enjoying the lakeside view, follow the lakeshore around to the left. Rising to an old dirt road in full sun, the trail reenters the forest at a map stand and easily skirts wetlands at the far end of the pond. Avoid the older trail, which appears to enter the wetland, and take the new trail that climbs a short hill then runs level above the pond. Slowly, mature hardwoods replace large pines. On the far side of the pond, an extensive pine blowdown requires some not-too-difficult tree-hopping.

As Island Ford Road once again comes into view, watch for a trail on the left before the overlook; it crosses the paved road. Climb the stairs to a low knoll. This trail quickly leads to the middle parking area at 0.4 miles. Watch on the right for the trail designated with a red blaze, which follows a tributary of the Chattahoochee River down to the river's floodplain. About 100 feet after you enter the forest, there is a pretty cascade in the creek on the right. After an easy descent, turn right on the main trail as it meanders along the riverbank of the Chattahoochee. Massive rock outcroppings and mature and old-growth trees abound along the banks of the wide, fast-flowing river. When you reach the first outcropping, follow the line into the river; there is a corresponding shoals churning the water in the Chattahoochee.

The forest opens up as you enter a wide expanse of the floodplain that has been converted to Hewlett Field. On the right are picnic tables and a grill. Continue along the river side of the field to a concrete launch and takeout point for kayakers and rafters. Next to the launch is a dock. Turn around and look across

Hewlett Field for a sign marking a path to the visitor center. After a thigh-burning climb, follow the trail as it turns left, then right, around the visitor center, returning you to the parking area. Continue past the front of the visitor center, turning right and descending along the same creek as on the descent from the middle parking lot. This time, as you reach the main trunk, turn left and cross a wooden bridge. With the Chattahoochee on your right, the trail follows the river as the hills on either side sometimes narrow the floodplain to a few feet. At 1.2 miles a side trail leaves to the left; soon after, there is a wooden bridge over an active stream. Once you're across the bridge, a second trail leaves at a hard left, as the main trail bears right. There is a large rock outcropping on the left with a corresponding shoals in the Chattahoochee on the right. A forest of American beech and oak follows an area of pine blowdown as the trail narrows and begins to roll up and down a series of small hills.

As the blue-blazed trail turns inland, a side trail continues along the riverbank down to a deep ravine. Return to the blue trail and turn left. Climbing into the watershed of the Chattahoochee, the trail is easy to moderate. Just before the trail dips to a stream, turn left on a gravel road, which rises to a pathway on the right 0.1 mile later. This loops around a forested cove with a stream running through it. At 2 miles the trail turns right and descends toward the river. Just before you complete the loop, the trail gets steep for about 25 feet and crosses a creek. Turn right and climb past the trail you just hiked, to a three-way intersection. The red trail turns right and climbs to Island Ford Road. Instead of following that path, bear left on the yellow trail, which descends into the Chattahoochee River Valley. Coming out on a low ridge, the trail descends a set of steps back to the river. Turn right and return to your car.

JOHNSON FERRY TRAIL

IN BRIEF

This trail explores a floodplain of the Chattahoochee River, including a forested wetland, then joins "the Hooch" for a hike along its riverbank.

DESCRIPTION

For more than 20 years, the Chattahoochee Outdoor Center was the summer fun capital for rafting enthusiasts in Atlanta. Each weekend thousands of people would visit the center, located at this hike's trailhead, and take a leisurely float down the Chattahoochee River to one of two takeouts farther south. They were forced to close in 2002 because of high levels of E. coli (an indication of dangerous pollution) in the Chattahoochee.

From the kiosk at the trailhead, follow the road to descend to a plain that was the parking lot for the Outdoor Center. The road soon changes from pavement to gravel and continues straight ahead. On your right is the return trail for the loop. Once clear of vegetation, the parking lot is in the early stages of natural reclamation. Black-eyed Susans and goldenrod abound in this full-sun portion of Johnson Ferry Trail. Look for the vestiges of humans—an overgrown picnic table here and there, an old tire, or a decayed sign giving exit instructions.

KEY AT-A-GLANCE INFORMATION

LENGTH: 2.1 miles

CONFIGURATION: Balloon

DIFFICULTY: Easy

SCENERY: There are some long-distance views of the Chattahoochee River and a forested wetland in the river's floodplain.

EXPOSURE: Full sun at the start and end of the hike, mostly shaded for the rest

TRAFFIC: Light

TRAIL SURFACE: Compact soil

HIKING TIME: 1 hour

ACCESS: Open year-round, dawn–dusk

MAPS: Map stands are located on the trail throughout the hike, additional map copies are available from the CRNRA main office at Island Ford (see separate listing), or visit them online at www.nps.gov/chat; USGS Sandy Springs

FACILITIES: None

SPECIAL COMMENTS: A National Park Service (NPS) map indicates that seasonal restrooms are available, but this is wrong.

Directions

Take I-285 West to Exit 24, Riverside Drive. At the end of the ramp, turn right. Travel 2.1 miles north on Riverside to Johnson Ferry Road. Turn left at the light, cross the Chattahoochee River, and make an immediate right into the parking lot for the Johnson Ferry North Unit of the CRNRA. Look for a brown kiosk in the center of the north side of the parking lot (opposite the entrance).

UTM Trailhead Coordinates

UTM Zone (NAD27) 16S

Easting 0739749

Northing 3758928

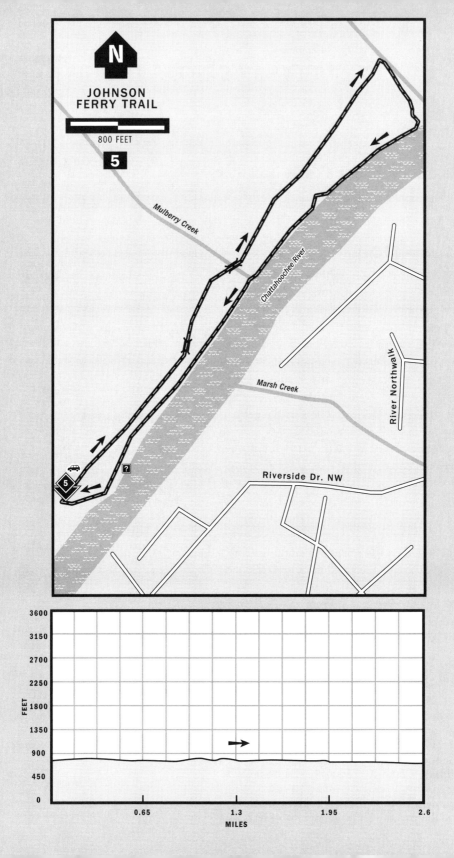

As you approach a bridge with a large Wildlife Viewing Area sign, the parking lot road loops to the right. Continue straight, crossing the bridge, and make an immediate left at 0.3 miles. Three hundred feet after the turn, a boardwalk first takes you across a stream then into an up-close view of the wetlands of the Chattahoochee River floodplain. Wetlands play an important role in a river's health. During times of high water, wetlands give the river a place to spread out and slow down, reducing downstream erosion. Also, they provide habitat for a number of small mammals and waterfowl and a breeding ground for insects, which the river fish eat.

At the end of the bridge, turn right. The wetlands, which are on your right and slightly lower than the trail, continue for about half a mile. They are occasionally visible but frequently blocked by trees along its edges. On this hike, the forest is made up mostly of white oak, beech, and an occasional sycamore tree. The area in and around the wetlands is mostly shaded.

Part of the hike is on a historic roadbed, which the trail joins at 0.6 miles, just after you pass two large post oak trees. The wide, nearly level walk is away from traffic noise, and the sounds of nature fill the air: a distant woodpecker tapping a tree in search of food, birds chirping to establish territory, and playful squirrels loudly crunching leaves and sounding like something much bigger.

Shortly after joining the road, a blowdown of some Virginia pine, courtesy of the Southern pine beetle, requires an easy walk-around. Finally, at 1 mile, a recently updated map indicates that the trail turns right. Several other trails in the area drew our attention—one ended at the CRNRA property line (marked by double red rings around trees), and the other two ended at a small stream.

Reaching the bank of the Chattahoochee River at 1.2 miles, the pathway makes another hard right, turning to follow the river back to the trailhead. Mostly shaded during this portion of the hike, Johnson Ferry Trail occasionally breaks into full sun for brief periods. When the trail is adjacent to the riverbank, there are some good long-distance river views. There is also a repetitive pattern on the trail: As it approaches each of the Chattahoochee River tributaries, the trail turns right, goes inland about 200 feet to a power line opening, turns left to cross a bridge, and then turns left again to return to the river. After turning inland the third time, the trail crosses the bridge at the start of the loop, and you are once again in the Chattahoochee Outdoor Center parking lot.

Continue straight until you see the parking lot road loop to the left. In the distance, almost straight ahead, is the brown fort-like building that used to house the center. As you approach the building, you'll see a narrow trail to the left at 1.9 miles. This takes you down to a Chattahoochee River access ramp that rafters and kayakers occasionally use. As of October 2004, the NPS no longer posts water-quality levels at the ramp because of a lack of funding for the project. From the ramp, turn around and face the Outdoor Center building. Walk up the ramp to the end of the cement, and turn left on a wide trail that swings around to the parking lot. Turn left and climb the paved road to the trailhead kiosk.

06 MIDTOWN ROMP

KEY AT-A-GLANCE INFORMATION

LENGTH: 7 miles

CONFIGURATION: Loop

DIFFICULTY: Easy

SCENERY: Urban landscapes, good long-distance views of the city from Piedmont Park and Atlanta Botanical Gardens, meadow-like environment of Piedmont Park

EXPOSURE: Full sun

TRAFFIC: Heavy

TRAIL SURFACE: Concrete sidewalks, asphalt pathways; compact soil trail in the gardens

HIKING TIME: 7 hours

ACCESS: Open year-round

MAPS: USGS Northeast Atlanta, Northwest Atlanta

FACILITIES: Full facilities at Woodruff Arts Center, High Museum, Margaret Mitchell House, Atlanta Botanical Gardens, and Piedmont Park

SPECIAL COMMENTS: Plan this hike around an afternoon show at the Fox Theatre, which is on the left on Peachtree Street as you return to your car.

IN BRIEF

This energetic hike takes you through the midtown area of Atlanta, passing the High Museum and the Arts Center, the Atlanta Botanical Gardens, Piedmont Park, Margaret Mitchell House, and Georgia Tech.

DESCRIPTION

The hike begins on Atlanta's first road, Peachtree Street. In 1812 Lieutenant George Gilmer left Fort Daniel at Hog Mountain (in present-day Gwinnett County) and began heading south along a low ridge east of the Chattahoochee River, building a road to the site of a Creek village known as Standing Peachtree. When Gilmer arrived, he built Fort Peachtree, the first building in present-day Atlanta. Over the years, Peachtree Road has been renamed, rerouted, and paved, but Atlanta's first road is still very much at the heart of the city.

From the parking area, return to the corner of Peachtree and 16th streets and turn right on Peachtree Street. The High Museum, on the right, is one of the best art museums in the southeastern United States. Opened in 1928 in the home donated to the Atlanta Arts Association by Mrs. Joseph M. High, the museum underwent major expansions in 1955 and 1983. Today the museum occupies the Meier Building, named for the architect who designed the Atlanta icon, but

UTM Trailhead Coordinates

UTM Zone (NAD27) 16S

Easting 0742149

Northing 3741575

Directions ⟶

Take Peachtree Street north to 16th Street and turn left. Travel 1 block to Arts Center Way and turn left. Arts Center parking, which charges a fee, is on the left. Return to 16th Street and Peachtree to begin the hike.

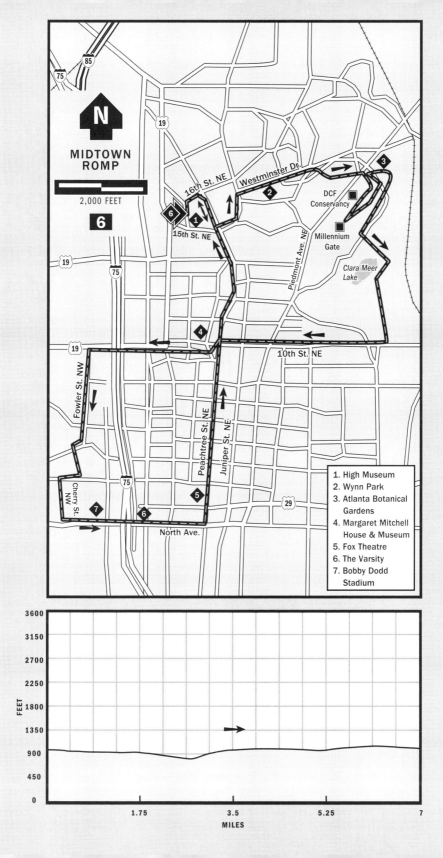

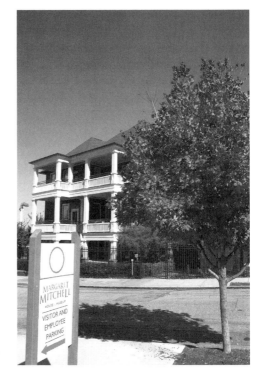

Margaret Mitchell House

in November 2005 the new 177,000-square-foot High Museum opened. You can visit its collection Tuesday through Saturday, 10 a.m. to 5 p.m., and Sunday, noon to 5 p.m.

Continuing on from the High Museum, you will see a sculpture, by the French artist Auguste Rodin, known as The Shade, and the impressive Woodruff Arts Center. Following a month-long tour of the capital cities of Europe, a plane carrying 122 members of the Atlanta Arts Association crashed on takeoff from Orly Airport in Paris, France, in 1962. The French government gave the Rodin sculpture to the city of Atlanta in 1968 in memory of those who died in the crash. Today the Arts Center houses the Atlanta Symphony Orchestra and the Alliance Theater in two buildings: one with a massive metal structure at the entrance and the other the 14th Street Playhouse a couple blocks away.

Cross Peachtree Street at 15th Street and enter the Ansley Park district of Atlanta, developed in 1904 by the Atlanta businessman Edwin P. Ansley. Turn left on Peachtree Circle, walk a block, and turn right on Westminster, where you come to the local gem known as Wynn Park. Not even a block wide, Wynn Park is one of the centerpieces of this community. Most days a variety of folks can be found enjoying the park, from young parents to older people. Playful dogs splash through a small creek, with a waterfall, that runs lengthwise through the park. Kids will have a blast here, whatever kind of outdoor activity they enjoy. At the end of the park, turn right onto the Prado, taking the north branch when it splits, and follow it two blocks, crossing Piedmont Road at a traffic light.

Across the street, at 1.1 miles, is the entrance to the Atlanta Botanical Gardens. As the paved road climbs, it passes a path to Piedmont Park, but for now it continue on to the picturesque Flower Bridge. Passing under the bridge, you'll see the entrance to the gardens on the left. After paying admission and walking through an atrium with pieces of Chihuly glass, wind your way right to the Dorothy Chapman Fuqua Conservatory. A variety of exotic plants and animals is housed in the climate-controlled rooms. The conservancy is open year-round but is closed Mondays, Thanksgiving Day, Christmas Day, and New Year's Day. Admission is $12 for adults, and $9 for senior citizens and children.

Return to the main house, exit, and once again cross under the Flower Bridge. Turn right at the marked entrance to Piedmont Park, taking the asphalt road that is closed to vehicular traffic. The road loops around the gardens, coming to the massive stone Millennium Gate on the right, built for the 1895 Piedmont Exhibition, a World's Fair type of event popular in those times. Make the first left, continue as the path bears left, and begin to circle Clara Meer, the lake that is the park's centerpiece. At 2.4 miles, as the road curves to the left, there is a small historical grouping of Atlanta's first streetlights (1855) and Atlanta's first pavement (granite blocks from Stone Mountain). From this triangle, follow the lakeshore as the path curves right and then swings left. As the path curves right at 2.5 miles, a second, straight path branches off, heading straight. Take this down to 10th Street and turn right.

This street begins as a hodgepodge of hotels, businesses, and apartments, but by the time you reach Peachtree Street they have been replaced with the massive urban structures typical of cities. After crossing Peachtree Street at 3.5 miles, you'll see a small, fenced structure on the left, looking out of place. The two-story dark red home with a white veranda is the apartment building where Margaret Mitchell wrote *Gone With the Wind*. Guided tours take people from the visitor center into the home where "Peggy" once sat at a Remington typewriter, weaving many of her personal experiences into a novel about the antebellum South and the changes that the Civil War brought. An informative display on her life and her role in the movement toward integration fill the basement. A museum across the street contains additional information about the book and the movie. The Margaret Mitchell House and Museum is open daily (except Thanksgiving Day, Christmas Eve, Christmas, and New Year's Day). Tours are given continuously from 9:30 a.m. to 5 p.m.

Continue west on 10th Street, crossing I-75/I-85, known locally as the Downtown Connector. This high-speed road predates the interstate system—it was a limited-access road that opened in 1952 and connected suburban midtown to the heart of Atlanta. As you leave the bridge, Alexander Memorial Coliseum, home to Georgia Tech's basketball teams, is on the left. Just past the coliseum, at 4 miles, turn left on Fowler Street. The campus of Georgia Tech is full of life on weekdays but normally calms down on weekends, except when there's a ballgame. Old-growth trees are common, and the campus is an eclectic mix of modern and historic architecture. Continue south on Fowler to 4th Street, turn right, then make your first left, once again on Fowler Street. At Bobby Dodd, turn right. The street climbs to Cherry Street, where you turn left. Follow Cherry to the Tech Tower on the left at the intersection of Ferst Drive and Cherry Street. Closely associated with Georgia Tech, the Tech Tower is built on a portion of the original four-acre campus. Return to Cherry Street and continue south.

At North Avenue, turn right, pass Bobby Dodd Stadium on the left at 5 miles, and cross I-75/I-85. On the left, just past the bridge, is a Georgia landmark, the Varsity. Known for its unique service ("What'll-ya-have?") and unique offerings ("naked dog walking"), the Varsity opened its doors in 1928, well before fast food became popular. At Peachtree Street, turn left and return to your car.

07 MISS DAISY'S ATLANTA

UTM Trailhead Coordinates

UTM Zone (NAD27) 16S

Easting   0744920

Northing 3739140

IN BRIEF

This hike explores Freedom Park—the largest urban park created in the 20th century, and a series of parks designed by the noted architect Frederick Olmsted for Druid Hills in the late 1800s. You'll also visit four major attractions: the Fernbank Science Center, the Fernbank Natural History Museum, the Jimmy Carter Library and Museum, and the King Center.

DESCRIPTION

Jessica Tandy won an Academy Award for her role as Daisy Werthan, an aging Druid Hills grandmother forced to accept an African American (Morgan Freeman) as her chauffeur-helper, in *Driving Miss Daisy*. The film depicts the changes that were occurring across Atlanta between 1948 and 1973 as Southern society became integrated. The movie also won the Academy Award for Best Picture of 1989; Freeman was nominated for Best Actor, and Dan Aykroyd for Best Supporting Actor.

The hike begins by crossing the road from the parking lot of the Jimmy Carter Library and Museum at the crosswalk to Freedom Park. The multiuse, interpreted paved trail follows Freedom Parkway and GA 42, which were built on the right-of-way of a proposed interstate highway that would have connected downtown Atlanta with Stone Mountain. Despite their having purchased the

----

Directions ———————→

Take the Downtown Connector to Exit 248C, Freedom Parkway. As Freedom Parkway curves north, GA 42 heads right, toward the Carter Center. Make the first right into the center and park immediately on the right.

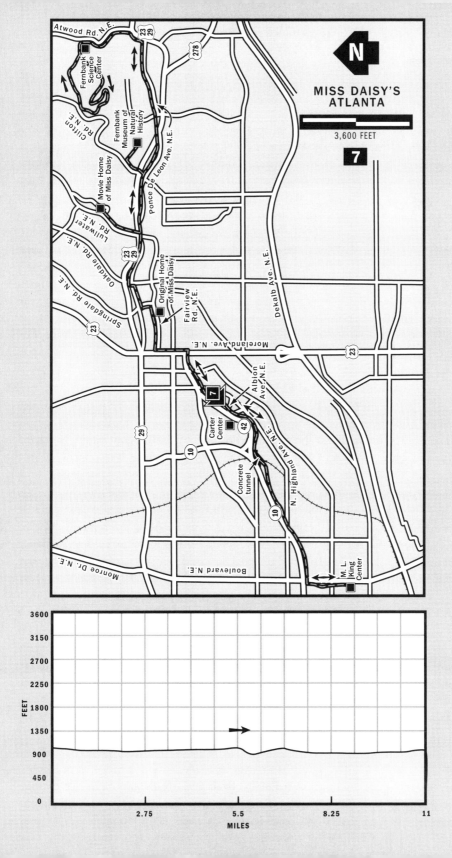

land and after destroying 400 homes, Atlanta, the State of Georgia, and the federal government were stopped in their tracks by a group of local citizens. The land was subsequently used for the Carter Library and Museum, Freedom Parkway, and Freedom Park, a 1.5-mile-long park that connects the King Center, Carter Center, and Druid Hills neighborhood east of downtown.

Where the Freedom Trail crosses Boulevard, there is a black metal sculpture of a silhouette of the Reverend Martin Luther King Jr. to introduce the King Center, a multiblock celebration of the life of Dr. King. The slain civil rights leader was born and grew up in the area known as Sweet Auburn, the business center of the large African American community in Atlanta. Turn left and walk two blocks south, then turn right on Auburn Avenue to reach the Martin Luther King Jr. National Historic Site visitor center on the right. Also in this multiblock exhibit is Dr. King's grave, Ebenezer Baptist Church, and King's boyhood home. The exhibit is open Monday through Saturday, 9 a.m. to 5 p.m., and Sunday, 1 to 5 p.m. Return to the Carter Center, but instead of crossing back to your car, continue straight to Moreland Avenue, where you cross the road at a traffic light and turn left. Walk two blocks, turn right on Fairview Road, and watch for 1284 Fairview Road, atop a low ridge on the left. Alfred Uhry based the character of Daisy Werthan on his grandmother, Mrs. Lena Fox, who lived at this Druid Hills address.

Continue on to Springdale Road and turn left, then make a right at South Ponce de Leon Avenue. On your left is Virgilee Park, one of the five that Frederick Olmsted incorporated into the main road of the Druid Hills community. Since the park's inception, Ponce de Leon Avenue has been straightened to improve traffic flow, but the parks are a lasting legacy of Olmsted's vision of the picturesque beauty created by combining natural settings with man-made features.

At Oakdale Road, Virgilee Park becomes Brightwood Park, which ends at Lullwater Street. Turn left, cross Ponce de Leon, and turn right, keeping the Druid Hills Country Club on your left. After crossing Clifton Road, you'll see Deepdene Park on the left. At the center of the park, a historic marker introduces the only original trolley station remaining in Atlanta, built in 1923.

Continue on to Artwood, where you turn left, then turn right on Heaton Park Drive. On the left is the Fernbank Science Center, a science resource center that includes Fernbank Forest, a multiacre, interpreted piedmont woodland that gives visitors an idea of what Atlanta was like before it was settled. Within its gates is a 1.1-mile, easy, loop, paved trail that offers a scenic view over the pond. The trail is interpreted, and maps are available at the entrance to the hike. The Fernbank Science Center is open Monday, Tuesday, and Wednesday, 8:30 a.m. to 5 p.m.; Thursday and Friday, 8:30 a.m. to 10 p.m.; Saturday, 10 a.m. to 5 p.m.; and Sunday, 1 p.m. to 5 p.m.

Return to Ponce de Leon Avenue and turn right. Walk to Clifton Road and turn right again. On the right is the entrance to the Fernbank Museum of Natural History, one of Atlanta's premier family attractions. Inside, dinosaurs greet you in an enormous five-story rotunda. Permanent and special exhibitions adjoin the rotunda on a series of balconies accessed by stairs or an elevator. Among our favorites is "A Walk Through Time in Georgia," which visits each region of the state in five interpreted exhibits and includes a dinosaur gallery of what Georgia might have looked like millions of years ago.

As you leave the Fernbank Museum, turn left, return to Ponce de Leon, and turn right. On the right is the members-only Druid Hills Golf Club. At Lullwater Road, turn right and walk to 822 Lullwater, the home used in the film *Driving Miss Daisy*. Set on a ridge (just as the actual home was), this home's exterior is featured in a number of shots. Turn around and return to Ponce de Leon, crossing at the light, and turn left. Walk two blocks to Moreland Avenue, turn left, and return to the Carter Center via Freedom Parkway.

Though four presidents have close ties to Georgia (both Roosevelts, Woodrow Wilson, and Jimmy Carter), only Carter was born here, in the small town of Plains in the southwestern section of the state. The Carter Library and Museum is the first publicly built library created to house the papers of a former president. Inside the library is a museum that follows the life of Carter from his youth to the present day. The museum is open Monday through Saturday, 9 a.m. to 4:45 p.m., and Sunday, noon to 4:45 p.m.

NEARBY ATTRACTIONS

Two Urban Licks is an upscale Atlanta eatery with a menu that changes daily, and everything we have ever ordered has been exceptional. Featuring good-sized portions of eclectic favorites served with nouveau flair, the restaurant is a popular New Orleans–style nightspot in the warehouse district near the Carter Center. An important note: They serve only dinner, after 5:30 p.m. From the Carter Center, take the GA 42 West exit. When Freedom Parkway bears left, continue straight one block and turn right. Follow the signs to the entrance.

08 PALISADES EAST TRAIL

KEY AT-A-GLANCE INFORMATION

LENGTH: 4.75 miles

CONFIGURATION: Loop extended by an out-and-back section along the river north of the Palisades

DIFFICULTY: Moderate

SCENERY: Best long-distance view of the Chattahoochee River in Atlanta

EXPOSURE: Mostly shaded

TRAFFIC: Moderate

TRAIL SURFACE: Compact soil

HIKING TIME: 3 hours

ACCESS: Open year-round, dawn–dusk

MAPS: At trailhead kiosk and on map stands throughout the park; USGS Sandy Springs

FACILITIES: None

SPECIAL COMMENTS: This hike includes the Fulton County side of Paces Ferry and the remains of an old building at the site of the ferry along the Chattahoochee River bank.

UTM Trailhead Coordinates

UTM Zone (NAD27) 16S

Easting   0737047

Northing 3752053

IN BRIEF

This hike follows a ridgetop as it drops to the riverbank at the Whitewater Creek entrance then easily climbs along the Chattahoochee to East Palisades. The trail leaves the river, climbing to an overlook before returning once again to the riverbank.

DESCRIPTION

From the trailhead kiosk, East Palisades Trail begins an easy descent along a gravel road through a typical piedmont hardwood-pine forest. As the ridge ends, the road begins a moderate descent into the Chattahoochee River Valley. About three-quarters of the way down, the road appears to end (it actually turns right), but the trail continues straight. Watch on the left for Long Island Creek, a large tributary of the Chattahoochee River. As you reach the level floodplain of the Chattahoochee, a side trail on the left that permits river access joins the main trail.

Bearing right, the trail comes to a second side trail, then a wet-foot crossing of a tributary of Long Island Creek. Turn right when the trail reaches an intersection. On the left is

Directions

Take I-285 to Exit 24, Riverside Drive. At the end of the ramp, turn left. Riverside Drive ends at 0.5 miles. Turn right onto Mount Vernon Highway. In 1.3 miles Mount Vernon dead-ends at Northside Drive; turn left. At 0.5 miles turn right on Indian Trail, which enters the CRNRA in another 0.5 miles. Travel 0.3 miles to the parking area. There is a second parking area after another 0.3 miles; to get there, turn right on Harris Road, then right on Whitewater Creek Road. The entrance is on the right.

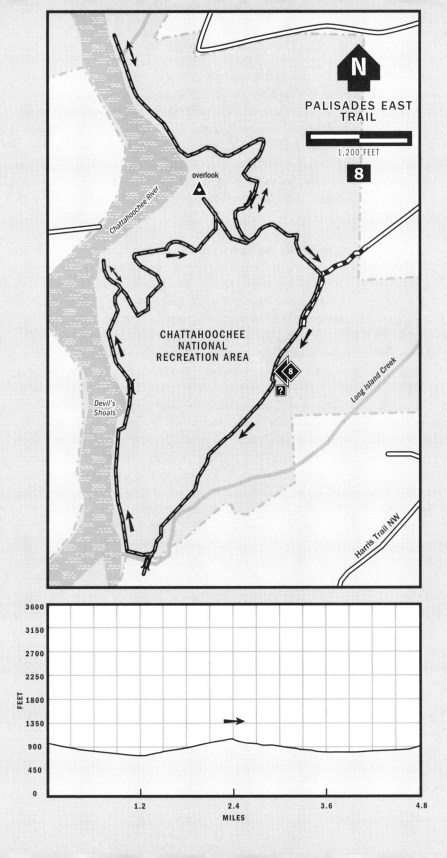

the new National Park Service bridge to the Whitewater Trail parking area. Spend a moment looking upstream from the bridge for a good view of the creek.

As you return to the trail, bear left. The trail curves to the right and joins the riverbank of the Chattahoochee. Enjoy a good view of the river, including its confluence with Long Island Creek. If you're lucky, you might even glimpse a great blue heron on this section of the trek. Out along Devil's Shoals you may see kayakers in a developed run on this section of the river, and you'll probably see larger waterfowl joining a fisherman or two in a quest for the Chattahoochee's noted marine life.

After Devil's Shoals at 1 mile into the hike, the footpath turns inland, easily rising to a slightly higher plain, and then bears left. At a tributary, the trail bears right and moves inland, coming to a T-intersection at a recently updated map stand. These maps, completely redone in late 2005 and early 2006, make it possible to change the described hike in this section that has numerous interconnecting short trails. Turn left and continue along the riverbank, approaching the Palisades. Take a few minutes to explore some of the rock grottos surrounding the path as it ends at 1.3 miles (the kids will love this) and return to the last T-intersection. Turn left and follow the footpath as it begins a moderate-to-difficult climb into the Chattahoochee watershed.

Beginning as a gravel road, the footpath becomes a winding, well-groomed trail as it approaches the top of the ridge. Once at the top, the footpath curves left and follows the ridgeline out above the Palisades then swings back right, ending at a gravel road with a map stand at 1.9 miles. Turn left and follow the road to the second marked intersection, then bear left, descending a set of wooden steps to the East Palisades overlook. This is the best view of the Chattahoochee River in the Atlanta area. Return to the map stand and turn left.

Watch for a trail almost immediately to the right and turn onto it. It follows the ridge briefly, then turns left at a three-way intersection and begins an extended moderate-to-difficult descent into the river valley. The trail to the right returns you to your car. At 2.4 miles into the hike, the trail curves right and steps over a small rise to a moist, level area replete with ferns and adjacent to a brook. After you step across the brook, the trail again rises, this time to a gravel road. Turning left and re-crossing the brook, you'll continue on the roadway to descend to the Chattahoochee. As the road begins to level, it reaches the river's floodplain. On the left, a rock wall enclosed a small, square area that once supported a fairly substantial building or bridge.

As you reach the riverbank at 2.7 miles, the trail turns right to follow the river through an area of massive rock outcrops. A few steps later, at a bridge over a small rivulet, is a second area of rock outcrops as massive as the first. This trail continues climbing near the river past a gravel road on the right and into a bamboo forest. After the trail winds through the large stand, it turns around at 3 miles.

Return to the three-way intersection at the start of the descent into the river valley, but instead of turning, continue straight on the gravel road. This brings you to the gravel road that leads to the parking lot. Turn right and walk 0.3 miles to your car.

NEARBY ATTRACTIONS

As you return to Northside Drive, turn right and follow it to Paces Mill Road, where you will turn left. This takes you through a decidedly wealthy neighborhood that includes the governor's mansion. Just before Peachtree Street, the Atlanta History Center is on the right. This museum has one of the best Civil War exhibits in the nation. The museum also has a section on Atlanta history, and one on golf legend Bobby Jones, and houses a collection of folk art from the Southeast United States.

09 PALISADES WEST TRAIL

KEY AT-A-GLANCE INFORMATION

LENGTH: 6.2 miles

CONFIGURATION: Double loop

DIFFICULTY: Moderate

SCENERY: Long-distance winter views, numerous riverside views of the Chattahoochee

EXPOSURE: Full shade on hills, partial shade to full sun along riverbank

TRAFFIC: Heavy along the Chattahoochee, moderate along the ridgetop

TRAIL SURFACE: Compact soil, gravel road, short stretch of concrete driveway

HIKING TIME: 3 hours

ACCESS: Open year-round, dawn–dusk

MAPS: USGS Sandy Springs

FACILITIES: Restrooms at the Paces Mill Entrance and near Akers Mill along the Chattahoochee River

SPECIAL COMMENTS: A helipad was added near the bathrooms on the Akers Mill end of the park for medical evacuation. When rafting was more popular on the Chattahoochee, many people badly injured themselves when they jumped off nearby Big Rock on the far side of the river.

UTM Trailhead Coordinates

UTM Zone (NAD27) 16S

Easting 0735974

Northing 3752749

IN BRIEF

The trail follows a high ridge to Rottenwood Creek, where it drops sharply. The footpath explores the riverbank and floodplain of the Chattahoochee near Paces Mill and Akers Mill.

DESCRIPTION

West Palisades connects Akers Mill and Paces Ferry on the west bank of the Chattahoochee River at Devil's Shoals. Little is known about Akers Mill, but we know quite a bit about John and Hardy Pace. John was a judge, and the first Cobb County election was held in his home. His brother Hardy ran the family mill and a nearby ferry. In 1850 Hardy was authorized by the state to build a dam across the Chattahoochee to impound water to power his mill, and his ferry eventually became both a bridge and a road. Hardy Pace, who died in December 1864, is buried in a private graveyard at the top of Mount Wilkerson (Vinings Mountain). The National Park Service has

Directions

Take I-75 North to Exit 258, Cumberland Boulevard. Turn right at the end of the ramp, travel 0.5 miles, and turn right on Akers Mill Road. Travel 0.3 miles to Akers Mill Drive on the right at a watermill. The entrance appears quickly and is easy to miss. Turn left at the signed entrance to Palisades West, then go right into the parking lot. To get to the Paces Mill entrance, turn left on Cumberland Boulevard at the end of the ramp, travel 0.4 miles, and turn left on Cobb Parkway. At 0.4 miles turn right into the Chattahoochee/ West Palisades/Paces Mill entrance. The road drops below US 41 and curves sharply left at 0.2 miles, passing under Cobb Parkway. You'll reach the parking lot in 0.1 mile.

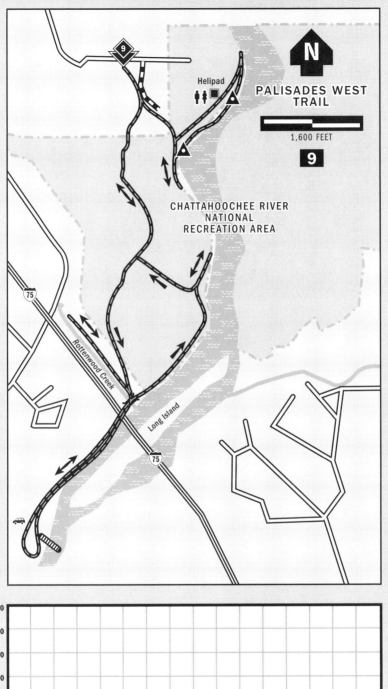

N

PALISADES WEST TRAIL

1,600 FEET

9

Helipad

CHATTAHOOCHEE RIVER
NATIONAL
RECREATION AREA

9

75

Rottenwood Creek

Long Island

75

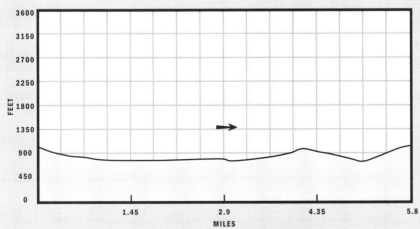

FEET				
3600				
3150				
2700				
2250				
1800				
1350				
900				
450				
0	1.45	2.9	4.35	5.8

MILES

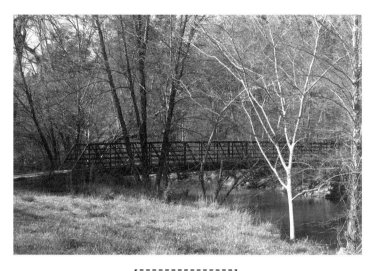

Palisades West Trail

proposed connecting West Palisades and Cochran Shoals (see separate listing) with a 0.6-mile trail.

As you hike from Akers Mill, the trail enters the forest at the trailhead kiosk and turns right on a gravel road where vehicular traffic is restricted. The road descends, at first gradually, through an upper piedmont hardwood forest composed of a variety of oak, American beech, elm, maple, and pine, mostly shortleaf and loblolly. Underneath the canopy, dogwoods, black cherry, and an occasional magnolia can be spotted. Continue on the gravel road, which runs along the first ridgetop west of the Chattahoochee. At a three-way intersection less than 0.2 miles into the hike, take a road off to the right where you see a sign for Rottenwood Creek. Follow this trail as it gradually climbs in full shade. As the trail bears left, a narrow paved path joins it from the right at 0.3 miles.

Soon the footpath bears left, only to make a sweeping curve back to the right along a mostly level ridgetop. Three roads branch off to the left in quick succession, the last being the road to the confluence of the Chattahoochee River and Rottenwood Creek. At Rottenwood Creek, turn right and explore the level plain of the river where the water forms some cascades and shoals on the recently paved multiuse trail. At the end of the concrete, turn around and head back along the creek side to a right turn on a metal bridge at 1.8 miles. After you cross, the trail curves left; there is a bench with an exceptional view of the Chattahoochee River on the left.

Curving back around to the right, the footpath passes under I-75 and follows the bank of the river to an open field at 2.5 miles. Watch on the left for a canoe/kayak takeout, which is the turnaround for this trail. Retrace your steps to the metal bridge, but instead of turning left, continue straight to explore the riverbank. The compact soil trail, which is occasionally in full sun, is rooted with repeated rock outcroppings that make this section of the hike challenging. You will pass a road on the left at 3.4 miles; the trail ends as you approach the tall palisade of rock 0.2 miles later. Turn around and make a right on the first road. The climb back to the ridgetop is a great 0.4-mile thigh-burner. As you reach the top of the ridge, the gravel road bears right.

At 4.5 miles you'll see a Rottenwood Creek sign on the right. At the next intersection, take the road on the right, to explore the Akers Mill portion of the CRNRA. The trail drops, and the next section of it is concrete. Take a side trail off to the right at 4.7 miles; alternatively, continuing straight ahead will also take you to the river. When the trail comes to a T-intersection, turn left. The trail soon curves right to join a gravel road; you'll find restrooms here. Straight ahead, across the surprisingly narrow Chattahoochee River, is Big Rock, a massive granite boulder.

Turn left to explore the riverbank, which ends at a sandy spot. Turn around and follow the bank to the Palisades for some excellent river views. As the trail gets rocky and harder to follow, turn around and return to the restrooms. Climb along the gravel road to the ridgetop then go straight to return to your car.

NEARBY ATTRACTIONS

Whitewater and American Adventures are great places to cool off after West Palisades. Whitewater, as its name implies, is a water-oriented attraction with a wave pool, Wildwater Lagoon, Runaway River, and the Cliffhanger (one of the tallest free-falls in the world). American Adventures is somewhat calmer, with bumper cars, a train ride, and small roller coaster. Return to I-75 and go north to Exit 265. Follow signs to the park.

10   PAPER MILL TRAIL

KEY AT-A-GLANCE INFORMATION

LENGTH: 3.5 miles; can be extended to almost 12 miles by combining with adjacent Cochran Shoals Park

CONFIGURATION: Loop

DIFFICULTY: Moderate–difficult

SCENERY: Views of the Sope Creek, which drops to the Chattahoochee River in a long cascade; remains of the Marietta Paper Mill, a mill on Sope Creek; occasional scenic views throughout the park

EXPOSURE: Mostly shade

TRAFFIC: Light–moderate

TRAIL SURFACE: Many rocky areas, especially near the river and tops of hills; some gravel roads; other portions are hard-packed dirt

HIKING TIME: 2.5 hours

ACCESS: Open year-round

MAPS: Throughout the park; available at www.nps.gov/chat and at the Island Ford Headquarters building; USGS Sandy Springs

FACILITIES: None in the park; however, this park abuts Cochran Shoals, which has bathrooms

SPECIAL COMMENTS: Sope Creek is named for Chief Sope, a Cherokee who remained in the area after the Trail of Tears. It is frequently misspelled as Soap Creek.

UTM Trailhead Coordinates

UTM Zone (NAD27) 16S

Easting 0736327

Northing 3758214

IN BRIEF

This historic trail offers hikers many options. Only the "main" path is shared with bikers.

DESCRIPTION

From the trailhead, descend a wide gravel road to the first path on the right at 0.1 mile. Watch for one of the new, more detailed CRNRA maps and a "You are here" arrow on a brown post at the intersection. This mapping system has made it much easier to hike these parks, and it is now in place throughout the CRNRA, including on Bowman's Island. If you hiked Paper Mill many years ago, please note that there have been extensive changes to the trails.

As you turn right, the man-made Sibley Pond is on your left, slightly below the trail, which traces the shore to the far end of the lake. Take the trail to the right as you approach a wooden bridge over a small creek to the left less than 0.1 mile later. The footpath climbs steadily to a ridge where pines have been damaged by borers, but in the new growth there is a wide variety of hardwoods and, for the time being, sun-loving bushes. The treadway begins

Directions

Take I-75 to Exit 261 (marked as GA 280/Dobbins AFB/Lockheed, with a separate sign for Delk Road). If you are heading north, turn right onto Delk; if you are heading south, turn left. Drive 1.4 miles to where Terrill Mill Road joins Delk. Continue 1 mile on Terrill Mill, then make a sharp right onto Paper Mill Road. Travel 1.1 miles to the Sope Creek Unit of the CRNRA. Turn right. The trailhead and pay booth are at the far end of the parking lot. The fee is $3.

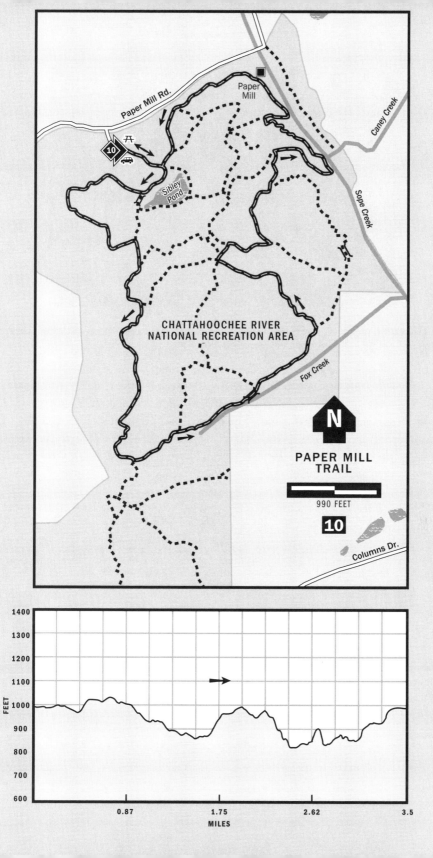

PAPER MILL TRAIL

990 FEET

10

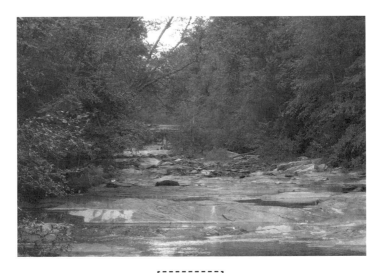

Sope Creek

to drop and turns right at a T-intersection at 0.5 miles. A few feet later, turn right as the trail rejoins the main trunk gravel road through Sope Creek.

Over the next 0.5 miles, the gravel road descends steadily, finally curving right at the bottom of the ridge. The main trunk continues straight ahead to Cochran Shoals Trail, but turn right. You will soon see Fox Creek beginning to form on the right. Over the next 0.7 miles, three trails head off to the left and climb toward Sibley Lake, but skip them to follow the creek as it grows. Continue straight, and at 1.7 miles the footpath rises and curves left, and a side trail leads off to apartments. The trail joins a wide gravel road 0.1 mile later, making the extended climb out of the Chattahoochee River Valley. At 2.3 miles turn right and follow this gravel road down to Sope Creek for a photo opportunity. Evidence of Paleo, Archaic, Woodland, Mississippian, Creek, and Cherokee tribes have been found near Sope Creek.

There are two ways to get to the paper mill from here. As you climb up the road that brought you to Sope Creek, a trail heads off to the right. This rocky, steep path is the only difficult section of trail in the park and should be avoided if you have a fear of heights, but it does feature more scenic views of Sope Creek, especially in winter. You can continue up the road to the next trail, which is slightly longer, if you wish. At the end of this section, at 3 miles, you'll find Marietta Paper Mill is on the right, down a steep embankment. For easier access to the ruins, take the trail to the far side of the Paper Mill Road and descend an easier embankment.

Built between 1853 and 1855, the paper mill was incorporated in 1859. Since it was built from rock, it was sturdier that other mills built in the area, including a gristmill and, later, a sawmill. Their raceways shared water from an upriver dam. General Kenner Garrard destroyed the paper mill and gristmill on

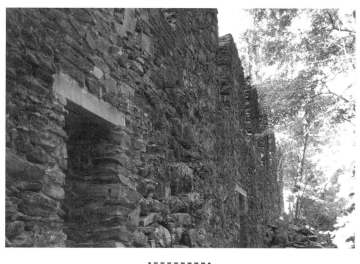

Paper Mill

July 5, 1864, as William Tecumseh Sherman marched toward Atlanta. Rebuilt after the war, the paper mill alternately flourished and struggled with the economy. It shut its doors in 1940.

Return to the trail near Paper Mill Road and follow this trail back to the main trunk. Turn right for a moderate climb to the parking lot.

NEARBY ATTRACTIONS

The Marietta History Museum details the rich history of the city and some of the mill owners in the Sope Creek area. For more information, call (770) 528-0431.

11 POWERS LANDING TRAIL

KEY AT-A-GLANCE INFORMATION

LENGTH: 2.3 miles

CONFIGURATION: Loop

DIFFICULTY: Easy, except on the climb into the watershed, which is moderate

SCENERY: Historic home site, scenic views of the Chattahoochee River

EXPOSURE: Mostly shaded

TRAFFIC: Moderate

TRAIL SURFACE: Compact soil and historic roadbed

HIKING TIME: 1.5 hours

ACCESS: Open year-round, dawn–dusk

MAPS: USGS Sandy Springs

FACILITIES: Restrooms

SPECIAL COMMENTS: Fishing is popular here, with anglers reporting some good brown and rainbow trout and shoal bass.

UTM Trailhead Coordinates

UTM Zone (NAD27) 16S

Easting   0736504

Northing 3754202

IN BRIEF

This trail explores Powers Island in the Chattahoochee River and then follows the floodplain of the river to a wonderful cove in the watershed. As you return to the trailhead, the path offers scenic views of the river.

DESCRIPTION

In 1819 the Cherokee signed a treaty with the United States that used this section of the Chattahoochee River to define the eastern boundary of this independent Native American nation. James Powers established a homestead and a ferry here in 1831. The Cherokee and local settlers gave Powers, who was a gunsmith as well as manager of the ferry and blacksmith shop, a brisk business repairing their weapons. When the Land Lottery of 1832 gave the Cherokee Nation away to settlers from Georgia, Powers moved west across the Chattahoochee River in 1833, to Vinings, in the newly formed Cobb County. He continued to oversee the ferry's operation. In 1903 the ferry was replaced by a bridge, near where the present-day I-285 bridge crosses the river.

Circle the brown Chattahoochee Outdoor Center, which has been closed since 2002, to reach an iron bridge with wooden slats that connects to Powers Island. Kayaks frequently run the course between the riverbank and the

Directions ——————————→

Take I-285 West from GA 400 to Exit 22, Northside Drive/New Northside Drive/Powers Ferry Road. As you come off the ramp, bear right on Interstate Parkway North, which curves left. Follow this 0.8 miles and turn right into the parking area just before the Chattahoochee River.

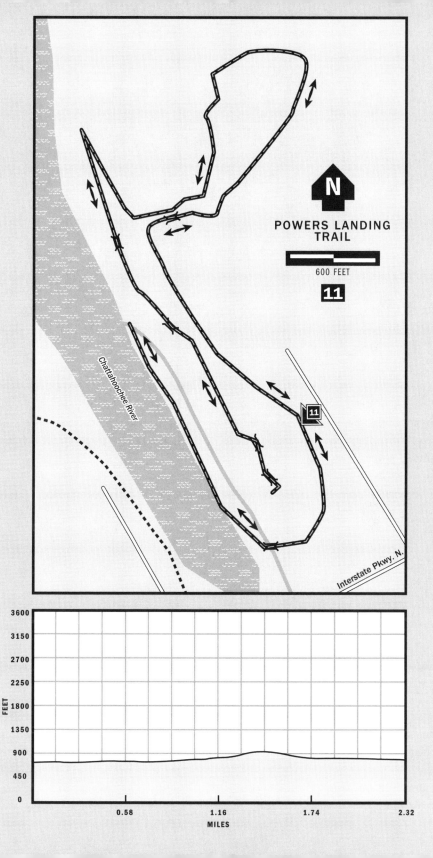

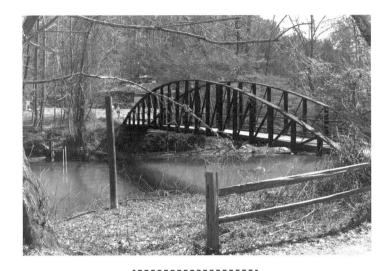

Bridge to Powers Landing

island. After crossing the bridge, join the footpath, which bears right, passing a canoe and kayak launch on the right, then curving back to the left and crossing the narrow island. When you come to a second launch site, on the windward side of the island, the view of the river opens up. Across the Chattahoochee is the popular Cochran Shoals walking trail. Descend the steps for good views up and down the river.

Turn around and climb back to the path, heading left at the end of the split-rail fence onto a compact dirt trail that follows near the riverbank. Passing through a mostly hardwood forest filled with large oak trees, especially close to the shore, the level treadway runs near the riverbank most of the way to the north end of the island. As you near your destination, the footpath heads inland to cross a small creek in an area of pine blowdown. Finally coming to a wide channel between two islands, this is where the trail ends today. Many years ago this channel did not exist, and it was possible to follow the trail to a deck on the north end of the island.

Return to the start of this trail and turn left. There are two entrances to the loop, but look for the one in the far right-hand corner of the parking lot. Beginning as a wide, level roadway, the pathway comes into a pine blowdown at 0.9 miles. After the blowdown, long poison-ivy vines scale large oak trees, and American beech trees abound. After you cross a culverted creek, the footpath reaches a three-way intersection at 1.1 miles. Turn right and begin climbing a narrower trail. On the left is a woodland stream. After you cross a wooden bridge over a tributary, the trail curves right, climbs a set of stairs, and swings left. As you approach a stone wall, ascend to a small level field that was once a homestead.

On the far side of the homestead is an old roadbed that was once a driveway. At 1.3 miles the roadbed heads right as the trail continues to climb to a ridgetop.

As a second trail heads off to the right, the footpath veers left and begins to climb to an unnamed knoll. From there, the path returns to the woodland stream, now on your left. As the trail descends, the rock outcroppings increase, and you can see wildflowers. After a set of wooden steps, the trail returns to the main path in the Chattahoochee floodplain. Turn right, continue to the next map stand, and turn right again.

Back on a gravel road, watch for a heavily damaged deck on the island just off the riverbank. The Powers Island portion of the hike once came this far north, but the changing currents of the Chattahoochee have made it impossible to reach the deck. The park ends in an area of large, poison ivy–covered trees. Turn around, return to the map stand, and continue along the bank of the Chatta-hoochee River by bearing right.

On the left, at 2.1 miles into the hike, a lone chimney rises, the building that accompanied it long gone. Feel free to explore the area, but watch out for small animals. Return to the path and follow the riverbank back to your car.

NEARBY ATTRACTIONS

This is a great Sunday hike because of Ray's On the River Sunday brunch. This upscale Atlanta eatery has been wowing diners for many years, and for good reason. The food is excellent, and the cost is reasonable. As you leave the parking lot, turn right on Interstate North Parkway and make a left at the first light, onto Powers Ferry Road. Go under I-285 and turn left at the light, also Powers Ferry Road. After you cross the Chattahoochee River, you'll see Ray's in an industrial park; take the first driveway on the right.

12 REYNOLDS NATURE PRESERVE

KEY AT-A-GLANCE INFORMATION

LENGTH: 1.8 miles

CONFIGURATION: Loop

DIFFICULTY: Easy

SCENERY: Multiple lakeshore views, forested wetlands, and a 17-foot-circumference white oak that was felled by a storm

EXPOSURE: Mostly shaded, except in the vicinity of the lakes and dam, where it is sometimes in full sun

TRAFFIC: Light

TRAIL SURFACE: Compact soil

HIKING TIME: 1 hour

ACCESS: Open year-round

MAPS: Available at the trailhead kiosk; USGS Jonesboro

FACILITIES: Nature center with native animals; restrooms, picnic areas

SPECIAL COMMENTS: There are many chances to see smaller animals, including turtles, tortoises, and a family of beavers, within the park. The nature center is open weekdays, 8:30 a.m.–5:30 p.m., and on the first Saturday of the month, 9 a.m.–1 p.m.

- -

UTM Trailhead Coordinates

UTM Zone (NAD27) 16S

Easting   0746166

Northing   3720877

IN BRIEF

Reynolds Preserve, with more than 4 miles of well-made hiking trails, offers an excellent family hike.

DESCRIPTION

William H. Reynolds Memorial Nature Preserve is built on the estate of William Huie Reynolds, a county judge who donated 130 acres of land to Clayton County to preserve both forest and wetlands for future generations. The preserve's board of trustees and the county have purchased another 16 acres of adjoining land that was once owned by Judge Reynolds for preservation. Within the boundaries of the park are the Reynolds home, a barn, other outbuildings, a number of ponds and wetlands, a large area of forested hills, and a nature center.

From the trailhead kiosk at the north end of the parking area, follow the paved trail through a mostly pine forest to reach the nature center. Among the pines within the preserve are loblolly, shortleaf, and white, although the white pines we noticed were all immature. Almost immediately on the right is the trail back from the Reynolds home. Continue toward the nature center. Inside are a number of interesting exhibits, including small amphibians and reptiles and an active honeybee hive. As you leave the center, turn right

- -

Directions ⟶

Take I-75 South to Exit 233, Jonesboro Road/ GA 54. Turn left at the end of the ramp and travel 0.9 miles to a traffic light. Turn left onto Reynolds Road, and travel 1.1 miles to the nature center's parking lot. There is an overflow parking area at 0.8 miles.

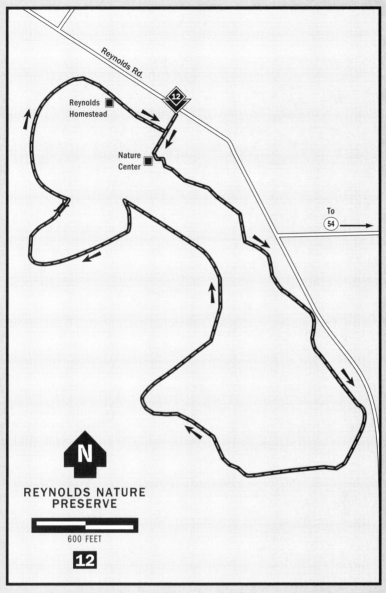

Reynolds Rd.

Reynolds
Homestead

Nature
Center

12

To
54

N

**REYNOLDS NATURE
PRESERVE**

600 FEET

12

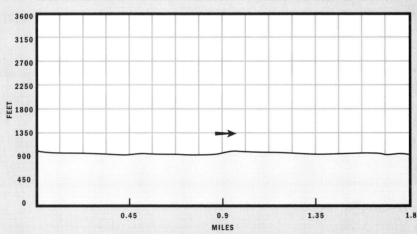

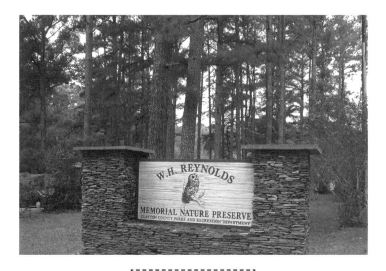

Reynolds Nature Preserve

and continue to a paved, wheelchair-accessible native plant garden adjacent to the nature center. The garden features plants like American beautyberry, Indian pink, and red buckeye.

Wide, level, and covered in mulch, Brookside Trail begins after the brick-paved native plant garden at a marked three-way intersection at 0.1 mile. It is the first named trail in our multitrail loop. Three hundred feet past this intersection, Hickory Stump Trail dead-ends into the footpath from the right. Continue straight on Brookside Trail to a series of three man-made ponds: Island Pond, Dry Pond, and Big Pond. Trails cross each pond, forming a dam built by local inmates in the 1930s, then they join Brookside Trail. On Big Pond, a dock allows hikers the chance to view waterfowl, amphibians, and reptiles from the lake. There is a large turtle population here, along with geese, ducks, and migratory waterfowl in the spring and fall.

Return to the trail and turn right, walk to the dam, and follow Brookside Trail to the right. There are some good views of the lakeshore to the right as you cross the dam. After the dam, the pathway becomes Back Mountain Trail, and High Springs Trail heads off to the right. Continue on Back Mountain Trail as it begins a moderate-to-difficult climb to a low knob in a piedmont hardwood forest of oak, hickory, sourwood, sweetgum, black gum, Southern magnolia, and tupelo.

Turn right at the signed intersection at 0.8 miles onto Hickory Stump Trail, a wide, mulch-covered trail, and follow it as it begins to descend the low knob; bear left at the bottom of this easy-to-moderate descent. Turn left onto the marked Crooked Creek Trail at the bottom of the ridge. When Burstin' Heart Trail heads off to the left, Crooked Creek bears right and enters an area of larger trees. The path wraps around a large white oak tree that fell during a storm a couple of years ago. After the oak, the path joins the creek that gives the trail its name. Along the creek's bank, the land has been heavily eroded from recent storms; English ivy abounds here. One upcoming project, according to Weekend Ranger Joe Ledoux, is to replace the nonnative ivy with a native ground cover.

Just past the area of erosion, the path climbs to a wide river plain and splits into two trails, with a third trail (Cypress Spring Trail) heading right at an unmarked intersection. Descend Cypress Spring Trail. After an unmarked trail on the left, which goes to another pond, Cypress Spring Trail splits as it enters a mature-growth forest. Take either footpath—they both lead to a boardwalk that crosses a stream in an area of large trees. As the trail curves right at 1.6 miles, the home of William H. Reynolds comes into view on the right; the barn is straight ahead.

Turn left at the end of the house, then walk around to the front porch. Originally, this was a four-room, two-story home with an enclosed staircase, the judge expanded the home, adding more rooms and an attic. Outbuildings include a barn and sheds, along with farm implements. As the trail leaves the homestead, it becomes paved. Portable comfort stations and picnic tables are near the trail in this area. Turn left at the next intersection and return to the parking area.

NEARBY ATTRACTIONS

A welcome center and the Road to Tara Museum are located in the railroad depot in downtown Jonesboro. The original depot was at the center of the Battle of Jonesboro, a pivotal engagement marking the end of the Atlanta Campaign. The present stone building, built in 1867, replaced the structure destroyed by Sherman on the March to the Sea. The depot is open Monday through Friday, 8:30 a.m. to 5:30 p.m., and Saturday, 10 a.m. to 4 p.m. Their telephone number is (770) 478-4800.

13 SILVER COMET TRAIL:
Mavell Road to Floyd Road

KEY AT-A-GLANCE INFORMATION

LENGTH: 8.6 miles

CONFIGURATION: Out-and-back

DIFFICULTY: Easy

SCENERY: Occasional overlooks into rural bottomland, although the area is rapidly urbanizing, and a good view of a creek from a trestle

EXPOSURE: Mostly sunny

TRAFFIC: Heavy

TRAIL SURFACE: Paved asphalt roadway marked with lanes

HIKING TIME: 3.25 hours

ACCESS: Open year-round

MAPS: USGS Mableton; map of the entire trail available for a fee in the Silver Comet Depot

FACILITIES: 3 parking areas with restrooms and phones

SPECIAL COMMENTS: Most popular section of Silver Comet Trail

UTM Trailhead Coordinates

UTM Zone (NAD27) 16S

Easting   0716257

Northing 3750648

IN BRIEF

Hike the level roadbed along the route of Seaboard Air Lines' Silver Comet, one of a family of trains that included the Orange Blossom Special.

DESCRIPTION

The Silver Comet was a passenger service train that ran on various railroads from Philadelphia to Birmingham, Alabama. The Pennsylvania Railroad and the Atlanta, Fredericksburg, and Potomac routed the train in the north and mid-Atlantic states, while Seaboard Air Lines routed the train on its track in the Deep South. Shortly after service was inaugurated in 1947, the train gained national attention when the

----

Directions ⟶

To Mavell Road trailhead: Take I-20 West to I-285 North, Exit 15, GA 280/South Cobb Drive. At the end of the ramp, turn left and travel 1.9 miles to Cooper Lake Road, the second left after the East–West Connector. The residential road winds 0.6 miles to Mavell Road on the left (watch for a sign on the right saying Nickajack Elementary School). Turn onto Mavell Road and travel 0.2 miles. Turn left into the Silver Comet Trail parking lot, which is adjacent to the elementary school parking lot.

Floyd Road trailhead: Take I-20 West to I-285 North to Exit 15, GA 280/South Cobb Drive. Turn left on South Cobb Drive. Stay in the left-hand lane. Drive 1.4 miles and turn left at the East–West Connector at a Home Depot Landscape Supply Store and a Marathon Station. Travel 5.8 miles and turn left on Floyd Road at the Quiktrip Station and Wal-Mart SuperCenter. Turn right on Floyd Drive, at 0.7 miles. Just past the Silver Comet Depot on the right, turn right into the parking area.

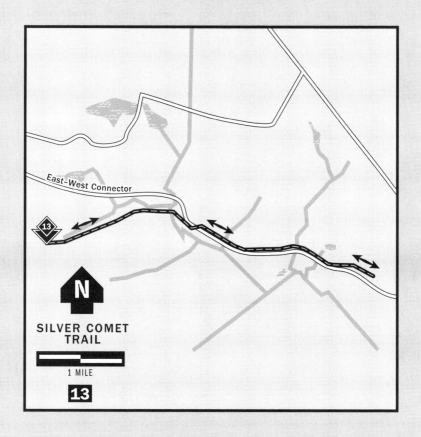

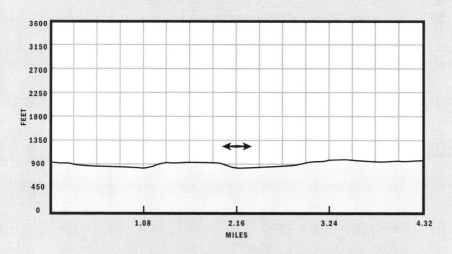

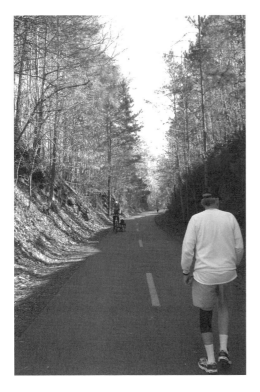

Dixiecrats left the 1948 Democratic Convention in Philadelphia and rode the train to Birmingham, where they nominated Strom Thurmond to run for president.

As competition from airlines and cars ended most passenger rail service in the 1960s, the route became a combined passenger and freight line before passenger service ended in 1969. After CSX ended freight service in 1988 and abandoned the track, it lay idle until the State of Georgia, three counties, and several state and local interest groups came together to build Silver Comet Trail in 1998.

Today the Silver Comet draws hikers, joggers, skaters, and bicycle riders from throughout the metropolitan area to southern Cobb County for an exciting day of sporting. Completed from Mavell Road to downtown Rockmart, the trail is on a railroad grade that never exceeds 4 percent. Some of the grade is uphill for an extended length near the Floyd Road intersection, but as you depart from Mavell Road, the trail descends slightly through a predominately pine forest with tulip poplar, pin oak, and invasive mimosa trees. Almost immediately, you'll see a side trail leading to apartments on the left. Throughout this portion of the trail, you can see homes, apartments, farms, and commercial establishments. Originally, the railroad bed was cut out of the rolling hills of the Georgia piedmont, then the debris from the cut was used to span bottomland farms. The Atlanta and Birmingham Air Line (a subsidiary of Seaboard) built the section of track from Howell's Yard (Atlanta) to Rockmart in 1904. An early example of these cuts can be seen at 0.3 miles, followed by the raised embankment of a railroad bed across bottomland.

There are additional improved trail-access points along the way, many from apartments and housing developments, but at 0.7 miles Fontaine Road Parking Area Access Trail comes in from the left. Just beyond that entrance, a sitting area allows you to take a quiet break from the busy trail. Just over 1 mile into the hike, Silver Comet Trail crosses a bridge over a creek.

A short distance past the 2-mile mark, the asphalt trail begins to rise noticeably, curving to the left and then crossing the East–West Connector at 2.4 miles.

This is one of the few places on the trail where the path does not follow the route of the original railroad grade. As you leave the trestle, the Silver Comet turns right, quickly regaining the original railroad bed. Shortly after the trestle, a side trail on the left takes hikers down to Heritage Park, where they can visit the remains of a woolen mill built in the 1840s. Hikers may want to explore a number of trails in this area, because the land is part of Heritage Park. On the climb back to the Silver Comet, watch on the left for a well-defined dirt road just before the asphalt path. Turn left on this dirt road and climb up the hill, watching for paths to explore on the left near the hilltop.

Once you have returned to the Silver Comet, turn left and continue walking west on the asphalt path. In less than 0.1 mile is a trestle over Concord Bridge Road. It is possible to see the Concord Covered Bridge on the left in winter and early spring. At the end of the bridge, on the right, is the paved access to the Concord Bridge Road parking area. If you want an up-close look at the bridge, climb to the parking area and bear right to reach the public road, then turn right. Carefully follow the road 0.2 miles downhill to the bridge, which was built in 1872. Turn around and climb the hill to the parking area and turn left. When you reach Silver Comet Trail, turn right.

Now Silver Comet Trail begins to slowly curve left, coming to a trestle over Nickajack Creek. Note that the old railroad ties of the trestle have been covered with wooden slats and paved. Following this trestle, the pathway begins an unusual, extended climb over the next 1.2 miles to the Floyd Road Parking Area. Passing a deep valley on the right at 3 miles, the trail passes under Hurt Road 0.1 mile later then enters a deep cut, which has been carved out of stone. This formation—rock, overlain with a few inches of Georgia clay—is typical of the geology throughout the piedmont and southern Blue Ridge Mountains.

Exiting the cut, you'll find a park bench at 3.3 miles. The trees, mostly older oak, are bigger here, although the forest is second growth. Walking along a ridge created by the roadbed, you will come to a traffic light–controlled intersection with Hicks Road at 3.8 miles. There is a small sitting area with a picnic table and park bench on the right at 4.2 miles, just before the trail intersects Floyd Road, which is also controlled by a traffic signal. Across Floyd Road on the left is the Silver Comet Depot, a bicycle-oriented shop with trail maps. Enter the Floyd Road parking area through a small sitting area adjacent to the shop, or continue 0.1 mile west on Silver Comet Trail to reach another entrance to the Floyd Road parking area.

NEARBY ATTRACTIONS

There are additional hiking trails in Thompson Park. Return to Fontaine Road and travel south 0.2 miles. Turn left on Nickajack Road and cross the railroad tracks; Thompson Park is on the right.

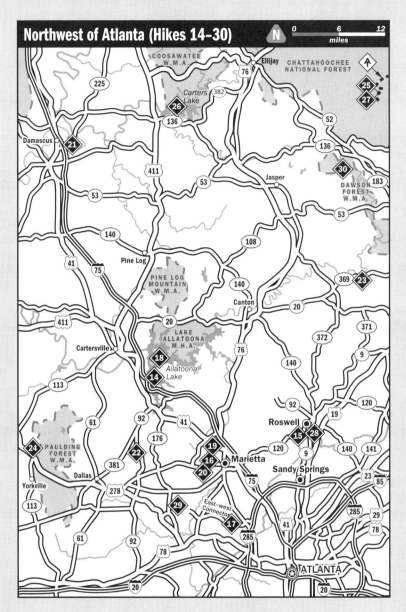

0   6   12
miles

NORTHWEST OF ATLANTA

14 ALLATOONA PASS TRAIL

KEY AT-A-GLANCE INFORMATION

LENGTH: 3.1 miles

CONFIGURATION: Out-and-back with 2 smaller loops

DIFFICULTY: Moderate

SCENERY: Allatoona lakeshore, with some excellent long-distance views; deep railroad cut

EXPOSURE: Full sun to partial shade at the lakeshore, shady near the cut

TRAFFIC: Moderate

TRAIL SURFACE: Packed gravel, gravel road, hard dirt

HIKING TIME: 2 hours

ACCESS: Open year-round

MAPS: USGS Acworth

FACILITIES: Nearest are Red Top Mountain State Park, one exit north on I-75

SPECIAL COMMENTS: Nearby Cartersville has a number of additional hiking opportunities. Call the Bartow County Convention and Visitors Bureau at (800) 733-2280 or visit them at http://notatlanta.org/hiking.html for more information.

UTM Trailhead Coordinates

UTM Zone (NAD27) 16S

Easting   0710747

Northing   3776937

IN BRIEF

Climb to the tops of two mountains separated by a railroad pass to view the site of the last Civil War battle in the Atlanta area. This trek includes a long, scenic lakeshore hike.

DESCRIPTION

Deep Cut, the local name for the pass, was built by slaves during the construction of the Western and Atlantic Railroad. William Sherman, who rode his horse through the pass in 1844, was so impressed by the defensive nature of the area that he avoided it during the Atlanta Campaign. On October 5, 1864, Confederate General Samuel French tried to capture the star fort above Allatoona Pass, along with the stores and munitions that were so desperately needed by General John Bell Hood's army. French returned empty-handed, and his group suffered 799 casualties.

At the start of this exciting interpreted trail is a map of the area on which the trail has been superimposed. Directly behind you is the Clayton house, a two-story home with a wide porch that served as a hospital for both the

Directions ⟶

Take Interstate 75 North to Exit 283, Emerson-Allatoona Road. Turn right at the end of the ramp. At 0.5 miles the road veers left, crosses railroad tracks, and then curves right. Do not take the road to the right before the railroad tracks. At 0.8 miles the modern railroad tracks are off to the right down a steep embankment. At 1.4 miles the road curves sharply right and enters a small community. The parking lot for Allatoona Pass is on the left, 0.1 mile after the curve. Go to the second driveway and enter. From your car, walk to the brown gate at the northwest end of the parking lot. There is a small path on the left-hand side of the gate.

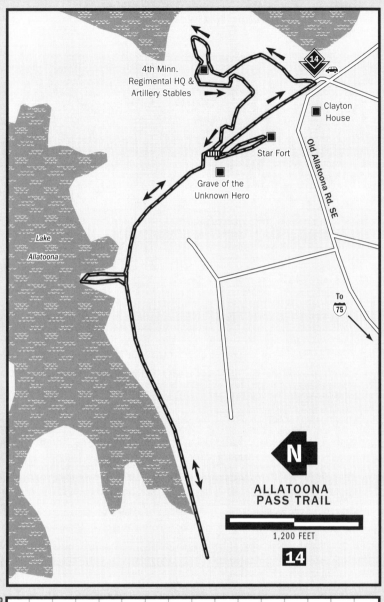

4th Minn.
Regimental HQ &
Artillery Stables

Clayton
House

Star Fort

Grave of the
Unknown Hero

Lake
Allatoona

Old Allatoona Rd. SE

To
75

N

ALLATOONA
PASS TRAIL

1,200 FEET

14

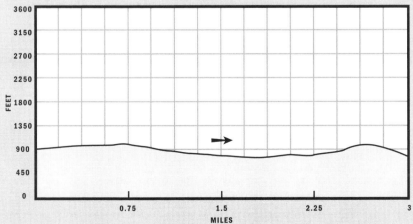

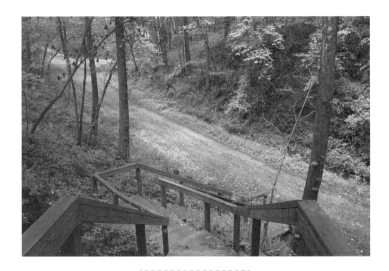

Steps to railroad pass

Union and Confederate armies. As you continue, the paved path turns to gravel as you walk toward Deep Cut, and there is an immense curtain of bamboo on the left. On the right are additional interpretive signs describing both the battle and the unique surrender demand.

From these signs, turn around and walk out onto a substantial, 15-foot levee built to impound the waters of Lake Allatoona. A chain across the entrance prevents vehicular traffic. As you walk the levee, the lake comes into view past Allatoona Marina, which is on your right. Return to the trail and turn right. Almost immediately, the pathway turns right again, descending to a small area dedicated to monuments from the states whose men fought this battle. Only Texas and Missouri have decided to mark the site—no Georgia troops fought in this battle.

Return to the trail and turn right. Immediately begin climbing a gravel road to the top of the mountain. The Tennessee Wagon Road connected the Chattahoochee River to Chattanooga. Allatoona, the small community at the southern terminus of the road, was a thriving railroad town at the start of the Civil War. Much of the town was destroyed when the U.S. Army Corps of Engineers built Lake Allatoona.

As the road climbs and curves left, you can see the eastern redoubt across a deep gully to the right. Built by Orlando M. Poe, this fort extended the defensive line for the Allatoona depot. Used to store Union Army rations, the depot and warehouses held enough livestock and flour to feed 100,000 men for ten days.

Atop the hill is a four-way intersection. Turn right and climb a flight of railroad-tie stairs. A few steps down, the trail splits into a loop. Take the trail to the right. This wide, shady, well-defined and interpreted treadway gives visitors a glimpse into the logistics behind a battle. The trail splits two more times. Each time, take the trail to the right, signed as the trail to the Crow's Nest.

Soldiers used a complex treetop flag system to communicate to Sherman's stronghold at Kennesaw Mountain. Flag systems were maintained for secret communications and in case a telegraph line was cut. During the battle, Sherman ordered the uncoded message "Tell Allatoona hold on. General Sherman is working for you" be sent, well aware that French would intercept the communication and be concerned about the presence of Yankees to his rear. Sherman, afraid the attack was a ruse to draw him out of Kennesaw, never left his stronghold.

Follow the signs to the eastern redoubt, where there is a wooden bridge over the entrenchments used to create the fort. A short wooden fence atop the earthen mound provided additional protection for soldiers. Turn right and follow the marked trail to the artillery stables. Turn around and return to the pathway. Turn left on the trail and continue to the Headquarters of the 4th Minnesota Regiment. Regimental commander John Tourtellotte was in charge of troops stationed at Allatoona before Union General John Corse arrived, just before the battle. Return to the four-way intersection and go straight through it.

Walk 0.2 miles for your first view of Deep Cut. Notice the two levels of the pass. Railroad workers removed the soft top layer, then slaves from local plantations removed the solid rock. As you begin to descend to the cut, there is a side path to the left. Two hundred feet from the main trail, the path overlooks a steep valley and begins circling to the right. Notice entrenchments on your left, used by Union forces during the battle. Rebels from the valley charged this Union line, failed to breech it, and retreated. Union gunfire from here caused many Confederate casualties in the assault on the star fort.

Return to the main trail, turn right, and continue descending into the cut. Approaching the bottom, the trail turns and dips rather dramatically, crossing a small drainage ditch on a stone-and-dirt bridge. Turn right and follow the level, shaded railroad bed 0.1 mile to the Grave of the Unknown Hero on the left. This was the original site of the grave of a soldier who died in battle. It was moved when Allatoona Dam was constructed, but for many years engineers on the Western and Atlantic maintained the grave. Return to the railroad bed and turn left.

At 1.2 miles most of the path is in sun as it begins to skirt Allatoona's lakeshore. A few steps ahead, turn right on a side trail to explore a peninsula of the lake. At the peninsula's point, you'll notice a pole with an extended flat top where an eagle has built an aerie. Scan the lake to see similar poles and nests. Return to the railroad bed and turn right. At 1.8 miles a gate across the road marks the end of the Allatoona Pass Trail and is your sign to turn around and return to Deep Cut.

Back in the cut, wooden stairs on the right at 2.6 miles begin a moderate-to-steep ascent that takes hikers to a star fort. A wooden walkway bridges entrenchments surrounding the fort's sally port (entrance). The Confederate attack came along a low ridge that is to your right as you step off the bridge. At the height of the battle, men from smaller surrounding redoubts retreated to the fort as the Confederates overran those positions. Imagine seven hundred men huddled within these confines, surrounded by the enemy, under fire, and running low on ammunition.

Take the wooden walkway to exit the fort, then follow the trail back to the steps. At the bottom of the steps, turn right. Continue straight ahead to return to your car.

15 CHATTAHOOCHEE NATURE CENTER TRAIL

 KEY AT-A-GLANCE INFORMATION

LENGTH: 2.5 miles

CONFIGURATION: Loop

DIFFICULTY: Easy

SCENERY: Excellent views of Bull Sluice; lake and river views

EXPOSURE: Full sun in the developed areas, mostly shaded elsewhere

TRAFFIC: Moderate

TRAIL SURFACE: Compacted soil, pavement in the developed areas

HIKING TIME: 1.5 hours

ACCESS: Open year-round, Monday–Saturday, 9 a.m.–5 p.m.; Sunday, noon–5 p.m.; closed Thanksgiving, December 25, and January 1. Admission fee is $5 adults, $4 seniors, $3 children ages 3–12, free for children age 2 and under.

MAPS: Free with nature center admission fee

FACILITIES: Restrooms, picnic tables

SPECIAL COMMENTS: Kids can enjoy a time at Camp Kingfisher during summer weekdays and explore the Nature Center on instructor-led hikes.

IN BRIEF

This hike explores the Chattahoochee River above Bull Sluice and then climbs into the watershed. The hike ends at the Discovery Center, where kids can learn about the natural world.

DESCRIPTION

One of the most frequent questions we get asked is where would be a good place to start if one hasn't done a lot of hiking. Chattahoochee Nature Center is one such place. Offering a deep-woods experience in an in-town setting, the nature center also has a number of natural-history and animal exhibits designed to keep the kids involved in the hike, and many of the trees and plants have signs identifying them. We normally hike these trails two or three times a year.

Walk through the asphalt-paved hallway between two buildings to a ticket booth on the right, or simply enter the building through a door on the right to pay the admission, then walk out the back door into an open area. Arriving early has an added benefit: large waterfowl can be spotted from a wetlands boardwalk. Turn right and follow the asphalt road down to a gated chain-link fence near a

UTM Trailhead Coordinates

UTM Zone (NAD27) 16S

Easting   0741751

Northing   3765541

Directions ⟶

Take GA 400 to Exit 6, Northridge Road. Turn west on Northridge and travel 0.4 miles to a right on Roswell Road, which crosses a bridge over the Chattahoochee River at 1.7 miles. At the end of the bridge, turn left on Azalea Drive. Travel 1.9 miles to a traffic light and turn left on Willeo Road. Drive 0.6 miles, then turn right into the Chattahoochee Nature Center and follow the road around to the parking lot.

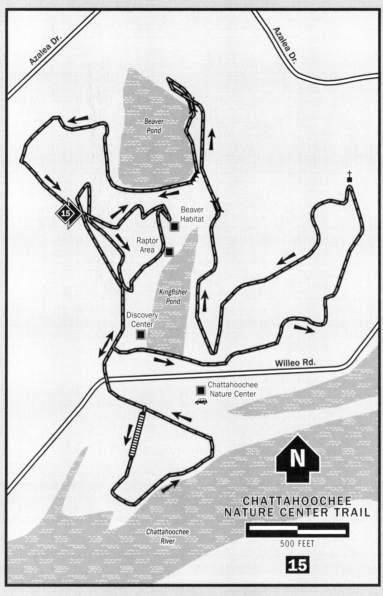

Azalea Dr.

Azalea Dr.

Beaver Pond

Beaver Habitat

Raptor Area

Kingfisher Pond

Discovery Center

Willeo Rd.

Chattahoochee Nature Center

N

CHATTAHOOCHEE NATURE CENTER TRAIL

500 FEET

15

Chattahoochee River

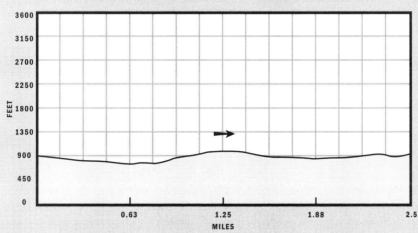

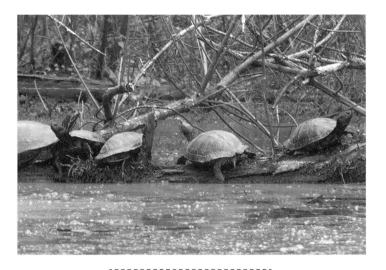

Turtles sunning at Kingfisher Pond

traffic light–controlled intersection at 0.2 miles. Cross with the light to a second unlocked chain-link gate on a boardwalk.

Jutting out into the Chattahoochee River and frequently in full sun, the boardwalk provides ample opportunity to study the unique wetland plant life in the area. Turn right at the first intersection and follow the boardwalk as it wraps around to the left. Bull Sluice Lake on the Chattahoochee River opens up on the right at 0.4 miles, allowing visitors to quietly watch some large waterfowl. On one crisp morning, we spotted a pair of ospreys, a great blue heron, and numerous smaller birds. Named for the waterfall that was completely covered when the lake was formed, Bull Sluice was created by Atlanta's first hydroelectric project, Morgan Falls Dam.

As you continue around the boardwalk loop, head down a short side trail on the right to an A frame–roofed area with seats. Here you can enjoy good long-distance views of the Chattahoochee River before the boardwalk curves around to the left again, where it explores an inland estuary. After returning to the starting point and crossing the road, enter through the chain-link gate and turn right almost immediately, following a concrete path down to an overlook on Kingfisher Pond.

On the left side of the lake is the Discovery Center, where instructor-led sessions allow kids the opportunity to experience various animals and reptiles. As the path continues through "Georgia's Living Wetlands," interpretive displays discuss protecting the fragile environment of the riverine wetlands or riparian zones. Water-loving trees, including river birch, black walnut, and water oak, have been planted to give visitors an idea of what a healthy riverine wetland might look like.

After a second overlook, a recreation Southeast Georgia's Okefenokee Swamp (complete with bald cypress trees), the trail splits. Take the trail on the right designated with red blazes. Called the Forest Trail, this pathway immediately begins to climb into the watershed of the Chattahoochee River through a fully shaded hardwood and pine forest. Watch for American beech and loblolly pine, which form a canopy over native magnolia (Southern grandifolia) and dogwood. A dirt road crosscuts the path where it jogs slightly to the right. A white-blazed crossover trail heads off to the left at 0.9 miles, but continue straight ahead to a Civil War–era grave at 1.1 miles. At the grave, the trail circles to the left, climbing to its highest point, where an orange-blazed trail intersects it. Bear left on the orange trail, which immediately begins to gradually descend.

After passing a white crossover trail on the left, you'll notice an old homestead on the right, made apparent by the home's chimney. After you pass a white crossover trail that heads off to the right, the orange and red trails end. Turn right on the blue-blazed Kingfisher Pond Trail, climbing to an interpretive area at 1.4 miles. A cutaway into the mountain, along with an interpretive sign, displays the layers of soil typical in the piedmont section of Georgia.

Bearing left at a side trail down to an amphitheater, the footpath once again begins an easy climb to a wooden bridge over a gully. Just before the bridge, a white crossover trail joins the footpath from the right, and the bridge makes a 90-degree left-hand turn. As the pathway swings around to the right, an orange-blazed trail joins from the right just before you cross a wooden bridge. Kingfisher Pond Trail ends at Beaver Pond. Bear right on the green-blazed Beaver Pond Trail, which follows the pond's shore as it easily climbs to a bridge at 1.6 miles. Just past the bridge, you'll see houses on the right; the trail quickly ends. Turn around and return to the three-way intersection with the blue trail, but continue on the green trail, turning right and crossing an earthen dam in full sun. On the far side of the dam, a concrete walkway joins the trail on the left, but continue straight to the end of the lake and bear right to the yellow-blazed Stone Cabin Trail at 1.9 miles.

The trail bears left at an open field through a forest that includes sweetgum and tulip poplar then descends gradually to the entrance, where the path is paved with concrete. Turn left and follow the walkway around to the right to reach the Bonnie Baker Butterfly Gardens. Plants in this area have been especially chosen for their ability to attract butterflies. Among the flora are blazing stars, Carolina silverbells, yarrow, purple coneflower, and the aptly named butterfly bush. Briefly returning to the green trail, the concrete walkway then takes a hard right to continue to a side trail on the right that heads down to a beaver habitat. After visiting the beavers, turn around and return to the main trail, where you'll turn left. The pathway leads through a series of raptor cages that house injured owls and hawks, and ends at a massive eagle habitat, where a pair of injured American bald eagles spends their time. Follow the trail as it bears right at the Discovery Center. Make a right onto the road, and watch for an old roadway on the right. Follow this road as it curves left to return to the entrance of the center.

NEARBY ATTRACTIONS

Roswell Riverwalk is a lineal park with many access points that follows the Chattahoochee River. It is currently 3 miles in length but is being extended.

16 CHEATHAM HILL TRAIL

KEY AT-A-GLANCE INFORMATION

LENGTH: 5.6 miles

CONFIGURATION: Out-and-back with a balloon at the end

DIFFICULTY: Easy

SCENERY: Civil War battlefield, with the massive Illinois Monument at the site of the heaviest fighting, entrenchments, and John Ward Creek

EXPOSURE: Full sun to full shade

TRAFFIC: Moderate

TRAIL SURFACE: Gravel road, compacted dirt, paved road

HIKING TIME: 3 hours

ACCESS: Open year-round; hours vary depending on season

MAPS: Available in Kennesaw Mountain Visitors Center; USGS Marietta

FACILITIES: None

SPECIAL COMMENTS: There are a number of interpretive markers throughout the hike with extensive information on the battle of Kennesaw Mountain. The paved-road portion of the hike has both markers and monuments and runs just east of the actual battle line in the area.

UTM Trailhead Coordinates

UTM Zone (NAD27) 16S

Easting   0722054

Northing 3758506

IN BRIEF

The trail follows a gravel road from Burnt Hickory to Dallas Highway, then parallels a low ridge to Cheatham Hill. After taking you to explore Civil War entrenchments, the trail descends to Kolb's Farm Trail, returning to Dallas Highway along a paved road. On the return to the trailhead, the hike leaves the main trunk and explores the watershed of Noses Creek.

DESCRIPTION

Sherman's Atlanta Campaign had stalled at the western side of Kennesaw Mountain. To the south, Confederate General Hood had prevented Sherman's favorite move, an end run around the Confederate line at Kolb's Farm. Now the massive army was sitting beneath the bastion of Kennesaw Mountain. Feeding the army was a logistical nightmare: Deep in enemy territory, some of Sherman's men were up to 8 miles from the railhead. Sherman decided to launch an assault against a broad

---

Directions

Take I-75 North to Exit 263, GA 120/Marietta/ Roswell, known locally as the South 120 Loop. Two exits head off the two-lane exit road before it rejoins I-75. You want the second exit, labeled Marietta/Southern Poly, which heads off to the right after the overpass. The road curves sharply around to the right before joining GA 120. At 2.8 miles turn right on South Marietta Parkway, which is also the 120 Loop. Drive 0.2 miles and turn left on Whitlock Avenue (GA 120). Turn left on Burnt Hickory Road at the Coldwell Banker and Whitlock Package Store, at 1.2 miles. At 1.1 miles the road enters the Kennesaw Mountain National Battlefield Park, and 0.4 miles later there is parallel parking on the left.

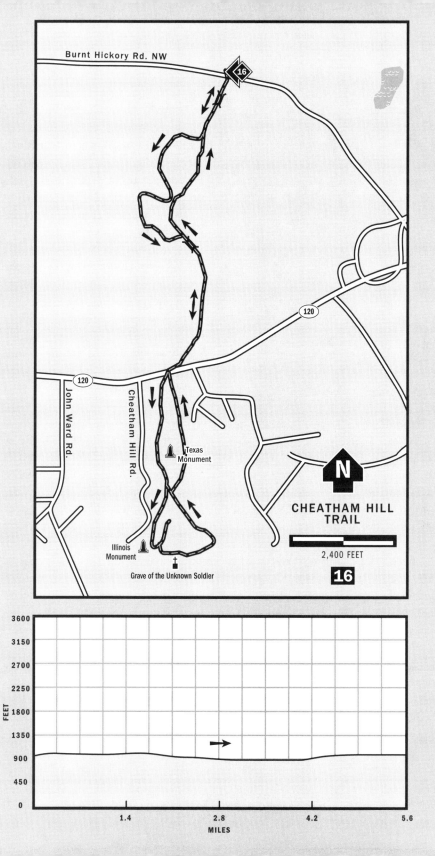

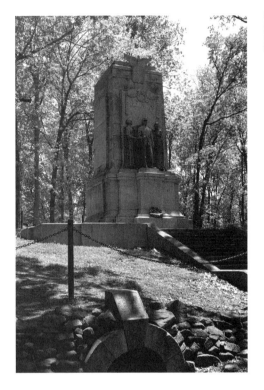

Illinois Monument

front stretching from the base of Big Kennesaw down to Cheatham Hill. He hoped to find a hole in the Confederate line—an improbable situation, given that his adversary was General Joseph Johnston, an expert at defense.

As dawn broke on June 27, 1864, the Union Army began the coordinated attack against Rebel entrenchments, starting at Big Kennesaw and quickly moving south to Cheatham Hill. The trail roughly follows just west of the main Confederate line from south of Pigeon Hill to Cheatham Hill. At the start of the hike, a field on the left just past a split-rail fence is where Union soldiers attacked a Rebel skirmish line manned by the recently transferred Georgia 63rd Regiment. The skirmish line was designed to warn troops of the approaching enemy. However, the men of the 63rd stood their ground against an overwhelming force. As the Confederate line evaporated, other members of the regiment charged, only adding to the carnage. Still, as the Union line neared the Rebels, it slowed, eventually withdrawing because the position became unsustainable.

On the left, an interpretive marker has additional information on the battle. After passing the first field, Cheatham Hill Trail begins climbing along a gravel road, with alternating cleared fields that tend to attract a wide variety of birds. The trail descends, quickly entering a pine forest (mostly shortleaf and loblolly) with white oak and American beech, a typical second-growth forest of the Georgia piedmont. At the start of the hike, there are some large post oaks; hickory joins the mix later on. At the bottom of the first hill, the road crosses a stone bridge then climbs as it curves, first to the right then back to the left. At 0.3 miles the return footpath heads off to the right, promptly followed by another side trail on the left after the last field. From this point to the Dallas Highway, the wide road runs through the forest but is only occasionally shaded.

At Noses Creek (named for Chief Noses, a Cherokee who lived near the creek), the roadway crosses the clear stream on a wooden bridge with no rail. Notice the stonework supports under the bridge, which obviously predate the current structure. Following along the creek, the gravel road begins an extended moderate climb in full sun to Dallas Highway. Be careful crossing Dallas Highway—the intersection has no traffic light, and people tend to speed through the Kennesaw Mountain area.

After crossing Dallas Highway, the trail passes through a split-rail fence, and immediately on the right is a sign indicating that Cheatham Hill and Kolb's Farm are straight ahead. After a short stretch through a mostly pine forest, the trail breaks out into the full sun of an open field, 50 to 100 feet west of the paved-road entrance to Cheatham Hill. On the morning of June 27, 1864, there was fighting along a line between where the path and the road now run.

Entering an area of a fairly extensive pine blowdown at 1.8 miles, the trail dips to adjoin the paved road at an artillery battery at 2 miles, separated from the traffic by a brown gate to prevent vehicular access. Off to the left is the Cheatham Hill parking lot, but the path continues straight ahead, and you soon reach an open field. At a four-way intersection in the middle of the field, turn left and climb to the Illinois Monument, a large, bold memorial to the men under the command of Union general George Thomas who were ordered to charge Cheatham Hill. After climbing the steps and viewing the monument, circle around to the left. There is an improved tunnel below the monument, dug by Union soldiers who were going to try to blow a hole in the Confederate line.

As you circle to the left of the monument, the path climbs to a series of Confederate entrenchments known as the Dead Angle. Hundred of bodies of Union soldiers who charged the Rebels were strewn in front of the entrenchments, but the Confederate line held, handing the Union Army its worst defeat of the Atlanta Campaign. At the top of the hill, turn left and follow the path along the entrenchments until you come to Mebane's battery, an artillery position that anchored the right end of Benjamin Franklin Cheatham's line. The hill was named in his honor following the success of the Confederate Army.

Turn around, keeping the Illinois Monument on your right as you follow the footpath curving to the left along the ridge. At the end of the ridge, the trail begins an extended moderate descent, passing the grave of an unknown soldier who was discovered by CCC workers who were improving the area in the 1930s. At 2.8 miles Cheatham Hill Trail turns left, joining Kolb's Farm Loop (see page 96) 0.1 mile as it continues to descend. At the second intersection, Kolb's Farm Trail turns right, and Cheatham Hill goes straight, quickly curving left and beginning a moderate climb to a parking lot at 3.1 miles. From here, follow the paved road that bears right and walk past a series of interpretive markers and monuments before crossing Dallas Highway.

After crossing the bridge over Noses Creek, turn left on a compacted-dirt path that enters the full shade of a diverse hardwood forest that runs between the creek on the left and a forested wetlands on the right. At 4.6 miles the trail turns right and begins to climb into the watershed of Noses Creek on a good thigh-burner to the top of a knoll. From here the trail begins a series of easy up and downs; turn left on the main trunk at 5.3 miles to return to the trailhead.

17 HERITAGE PARK TRAIL

KEY AT-A-GLANCE INFORMATION

LENGTH: 3.5 miles

CONFIGURATION: Out-and-back

DIFFICULTY: Easy

SCENERY: This trail features great riverside views most of the way, rising near the end to afford an excellent "above it all" view. There are historic buildings near the trail.

EXPOSURE: Shaded, except for the initial 0.3 miles, which is in full sun

TRAFFIC: Moderate

TRAIL SURFACE: Gravel road turning to packed dirt at the end

HIKING TIME: 2.5 hours

ACCESS: Open year-round

MAPS: USGS Mableton

FACILITIES: Restrooms are available at the visitor center at the start of the hike; there are picnic tables along the hike.

SPECIAL COMMENTS: This area developed into an industrial center because of water power and the nearby Western and Atlantic Railroad.

IN BRIEF

This historic road explores a portion of Confederate general Joseph Johnston's Smyrna Line and the remains of an old woolen mill. Hikers can view Ruff's Mill and continue on to see Concord Covered Bridge.

DESCRIPTION

From the parking lot, walk toward the stone and wood interpretive center. Here there is detailed information on the historic sites along the trail in addition to a viewing platform that overlooks the wetland marsh formed by Nickajack Creek. From the building, walk to the northwest corner of the parking area, where the trail enters the woods and gradually descends a compacted-soil trail. After an S-curve at the start of the treadway, two immense beech trees on either side of the path shade the area. A small overlook allows you to inspect the lower beech tree.

Next, the path gradually declines to a marsh that is traversed by a wooden boardwalk. It's easy to spot various smaller wetland birds here. About 200 feet farther along, a more substantial iron bridge with wooden planking carries you across Nickajack Creek. Look to the left as you cross and you'll see water cascading over shoals. Immediately after

UTM Trailhead Coordinates

UTM Zone (NAD27)   16S

Easting   0727323

Northing   3746836

Directions

Take I-20 West to Exit 51B (I-285 North). Travel north to South Cobb Drive (Exit 15). At the end of the ramp, turn left and drive 1.3 miles to the East–West Connector. Turn left and get in the left-hand lane. Fontaine Road heads off to the left at 2.5 miles. After turning left, travel 0.4 miles to the entrance to Heritage Park on the right. Follow the parking lot around to the far side of the visitor center.

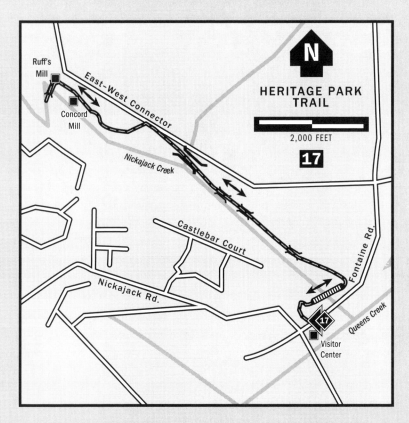

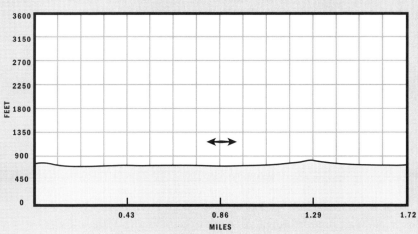

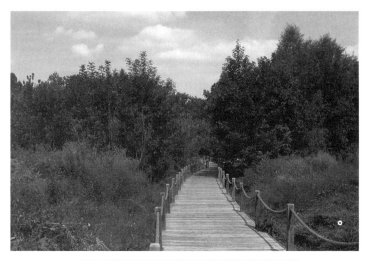

Boardwalk over Nickajack Creek Wetlands

the end of the bridge, turn left at an unmarked intersection of four trails.

Now a gravel road, the trail begins to parallel Nickajack Creek on the left. Following the battle of Kennesaw Mountain, confederate General Joseph Johnston pulled back to a secondary defensive position known as the Smyrna Line. Nickajack Creek formed the southern end of the line. Soldiers stationed on this part of the trail on July 3, 1864, came under artillery fire in the morning. This was the only fighting in this vicinity.

First in a series of scenic creekside shots comes into view at 0.4 miles. Photographers will want to get here before noon for the best pictures. Shortly past the scenic view, houses are visible across the creek and up a hill. At 0.5 miles the trail crosses the first of a string of small wooden bridges across tributaries of Nickajack Creek. Immediately after the first bridge, there is a side trail to the right. The bridge at 1.1 miles is longer than the others, spanning a creek, a wetland area, and another creek. On an early-fall morning, it is possible to see a number of large waterfowl in this area.

About 0.2 miles after the wetlands, the pathway makes an abrupt left turn, and the traffic noise grows very loud. At this point, the East–West Connector, a major Cobb County thoroughfare, is up the embankment to the right. A few steps past the turn is a picnic table, and just beyond the table is an excellent view of the creek. The far riverbank is a wall of river-worn granite, common in the Georgia piedmont. As you continue down the treadway, the traffic noise subsides. At 1.6 miles the historic woolen mill comes into view.

The water from Nickajack Creek powered Concord Woolen Mills, a three-story building made of fieldstone and cement. Today only a portion of the mill remains. Built before the Civil War by Robert Daniel and Martin Ruff, the mill produced wool for the Confederacy and was among Sherman's targets during the

Atlanta Campaign. Union soldiers destroyed it in 1864 shortly after they captured it. Following the war, the mill incorporated and was rebuilt. In 1872 the western Georgia industrialist Seaborn Love and others purchased the mill and a portion of the surrounding land that included housing for mill workers.

In 1910 Annie (Gillespie) Johnson tried to bring in Russian Jews who were part of the Galveston movement to revitalize the mill. Unfortunately, her request for help was rejected; the mill was abandoned and fell into disrepair. When the East–West Connector and the nearby Silver Comet Trail were built, metal supports were added to what remained of the building to ensure that blasting would not further damage the walls. Take time to explore the woolen mill and an adjacent outbuilding.

Returning to the path, you'll find two unmarked paved trails heading off to the right as you pass the mill. These connect Heritage Park to Silver Comet Trail, a mixed-use paved trail. As you continue, the path begins to slowly and steadily rise; there are a number of side trails to both the left and the right. At 1.7 miles there is a long-distance view from the trail, which is now 100 feet above Nickajack Creek. Five hundred feet farther on, the trail makes a hard left turn and begins an easy descent to Ruff's Mill and Concord Bridge.

Known as Daniel and Ruff Mill when it was built before the Civil War, by the time Sherman's troops arrived in 1864 the mill was known simply as Ruff's Mill. Unlike the woolen mill, Ruff's gristmill survived the Yankee invasion and prospered after the war, eventually being sold and run as Martin's Feed and Grain. When Asbury Martin left, he moved lock, stock, and millworks to another site, so all that is left is the mill building, along with the miller's house, both of which are privately owned.

At the roadway, turn left and walk down about 100 feet to the Concord Covered Bridge. One of the shorter remaining covered bridges in Georgia, Concord spans 130 feet between two stone abutments. Two modern concrete piers give the heavily used covered bridge additional support in the center. This 1872 bridge features queen post trusses and was completely renovated in 1983.

An earlier structure spanned Nickajack Creek in this spot as early as 1848. On July 3, 1864, Confederate soldiers stationed on high ground just south of the bridge came under Union attack. They were driven from the ridge, crossed Concord Bridge, and reformed a line on the north side of Nickajack Creek. The following day, the battle of Ruff's Mill was fought about a mile and a half from the mill.

This is the end of the hike. Turn around and retrace your steps to the car.

NEARBY ATTRACTIONS

The Silver Comet Trail (see hike 13 and hike 24) that connects to Heritage Park at Concord Woolen Mill is a paved, multiuse trail open every day from dawn to dusk.

18 HOMESTEAD TRAIL

KEY AT-A-GLANCE INFORMATION

LENGTH: 5.7 miles

CONFIGURATION: Balloon

DIFFICULTY: Easy

SCENERY: Multiple views of Lake Allatoona and its tributaries

EXPOSURE: Mostly shaded

TRAFFIC: Moderate

TRAIL SURFACE: Mulched, compacted soil with few rocks or roots

HIKING TIME: 3 hours

ACCESS: Daily, 7 a.m.–10 p.m.

MAPS: Handout available at trailhead and in visitor center

FACILITIES: Restrooms at trailhead

SPECIAL COMMENTS: Red Top Mountain is a popular stop in the Georgia State Park system, with a lodge and restaurant, multiple hiking trails, a marina, and a beach.

- -

UTM Trailhead Coordinates

UTM Zone (NAD27) 16S

Easting 0711360

Northing 3780759

IN BRIEF

This hike explores a peninsula of Lake Allatoona and the lake's watershed.

DESCRIPTION

Red Top Mountain State Park lies on a peninsula that was slated to be part of I-75, but local residents strongly objected to the destruction of this beautiful area, so the state and federal governments rerouted I-75 to the west and preserved the state park. The name Red Top comes from the presence of iron in the Georgia clay. Today, in addition to 12 miles of hiking trails, the 1,562-acre park contains a lodge and conference center, camping and RV sites, a beach (in season), a boating dock, picnic areas, and group shelters.

Homestead Trail begins in front of the visitor center, heading off on the left as you approach the building. A few steps down the path, you'll find a trailhead kiosk with information about the park and some of the animals you may see on your journey. The path soon passes a ranger residence and a side trail to a group shelter, both on the left side of the path as it continues to drop into a valley through a fair few trees with southern pine beetle damage.

Just short of 0.4 miles, Sweet Gum Trail heads off to the right at a marked intersection. Between the visitor center and the road to the lodge, Sweet Gum Trail and Homestead Trail run parallel. Normally separated by a valley,

- -

Directions ———————————————▶

Take I-75 North to Exit 285, Red Top Mountain Road. At the end of the ramp, turn right and travel 1.8 miles to the visitor center.

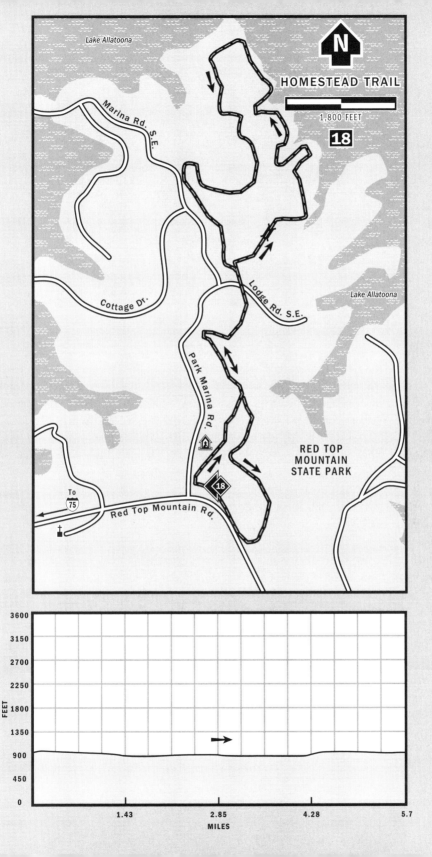

HOMESTEAD TRAIL

N

1,800 FEET

18

Lake Allatoona

Marina Rd. S.E.

Cottage Dr.

Lodge Rd. S.E.

Lake Allatoona

Park Marina Rd.

RED TOP
MOUNTAIN
STATE PARK

To **75**

18

Red Top Mountain Rd.

FEET

3600
3150
2700
2250
1800
1350
900
450
0

1.43   2.85   4.28   5.7
MILES

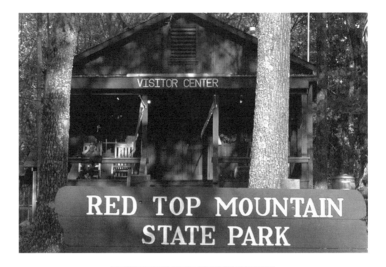

Visitor Center at Red Top Mountain

they share the path for 200 feet here. Sweet Gum Trail bears right at a sign that says simply "Lodge."

Once Sweet Gum Trail leaves, Homestead Trail makes a U-turn, rises at an easy-to-moderate grade, and then makes a second U-turn. As the treadway follows the curve of the hill around to the left, you'll begin to notice orange blazes and interpretive signs. Just past a boardwalk over a wet area, the footpath makes an easy climb to and across Lodge Road. Just after the road, a second lodge trail heads off to the right as Homestead Trail descends to the start of the loop.

The loop can be hiked in either direction, but we chose to walk it counterclockwise because a small hiker sign had an arrow pointing that way. Skirting a valley on the right, the treadway passes the lodge's wastewater-treatment plant, which is on the right-hand side of the path. Watch for an area of impressive sweetgum trees near the plant. The sweetgum tree was important to the Cherokee who inhabited the area before the settlers moved in. They chewed the hardened resin of the tree, and they boiled the fruits and leaves to make a medicinal tea. They also mixed the gum with beef tallow to create a salve for wounds.

A tributary of the Etowah River forms on the right as the trail gradually descends. The valley begins to widen and the number of rock outcroppings increases, but the trail curves left and heads away from the creek. As the path turns right, it crosses a bridge, then returns to the tributary, which now has taken on the appearance of a dry lake bottom. When Lake Allatoona is full, this should be a shallow arm. As you continue around the side of the mountain to the left, Lake Allatoona comes into full view at 1.4 miles.

Proposed in the 1930s, the construction of Lake Allatoona began in 1941, only to be delayed by World War II. Built as a watershed lake, Allatoona was designed to hold back the waters of the Etowah River that had regularly flooded the city of Rome, Georgia. During the fall and winter, when rainfall is at its lowest, the lake is partially drained. Spring rains fill the lake instead of inundating the relatively flat land of the Etowah River Valley. In 1947, only months before the dam was complete, the Etowah flooded for the last time.

Coming out on the first peninsula at 1.6 miles, Homestead Trail gently curves left. Returning to a cove, the pathway crosses a rivulet on a wooden bridge and then returns down another finger of the lake. This pattern will be repeated throughout the lake portion of the hike. About halfway through the second peninsula, there are a number of rock outcroppings, and the number and size of nearby boulders increases. A few feet past the 2-mile marker a trail on the right descends a moderate slope to the lakeshore. After passing this side trail, the main trail turns in to a cove, makes another U-turn, and returns to the lake. Now making an extended run alongside but above the lake, the trail gently curves left and begins to climb away from the lake. At 2.7 miles a blue-blazed trail heads off Homestead Trail on the right, running toward the lake. This is the final access point to the lake on the pathway.

Running inland, the trail makes easy-to-moderate up-and-down climbs, normally ascending 50 feet or so before falling by about the same amount. As the trail climbs to 3.5 miles, a blue-blazed trail heads off to the left. Take just a few more steps, and Homestead Trail curves right and begins to descend into a valley. The treadway also becomes somewhat rocky for the first time. As it begins climbing, Homestead Trail winds to the left, rising and straightening as it nears the top of the mountain. Look down on the left, and you will see the trail you walked earlier. From this point, it's an easy walk to the start of the loop. Turn right and continue down the trail to the second intersection with Sweet Gum Trail, at 4.9 miles. Homestead Trail curves to the right as Sweet Gum Trail goes straight before bearing left, then paralleling Homestead Trail on the other side of a valley. At 5.2 miles Sweet Gum Trail reaches a four-way intersection. Turn left onto the visitor center loop. This easy return trail is a slightly longer return route to the Red Top Mountain visitor center parking lot. After it curves around to an overlook, the trail continues a moderate climb through a boulder field to Red Top Mountain Road. Turn right and return to the trailhead parking lot.

NEARBY ATTRACTIONS

Cartersville is home to the world-class Booth Western Art Museum. One of the finest collections of Western and Civil War art, the Booth Museum also has an exhibit on the presidents of the United States that features a brief biography, a photograph or painting, and a signed sample of each man's handwriting. Take I-75 North to Exit 288, Main Street. Turn left and travel 2.3 miles. Turn left at Wall Street and follow the signs for two blocks to the parking area.

19 KENNESAW MOUNTAIN: BURNT HICKORY LOOP

KEY AT-A-GLANCE INFORMATION

LENGTH: 5 miles

CONFIGURATION: Loop

DIFFICULTY: Difficult

SCENERY: 360-degree views, including Atlanta and Stone Mountain to the east; Pine Mountain, Lost Mountain, and the mountains of Georgia's Valley and Ridge section to the west and northwest; and the Allatoona Mountains to the north

EXPOSURE: Mostly shaded, except on peaks, where the trail is in full sun

TRAFFIC: Heavy, especially on the first mile

TRAIL SURFACE: Rocky soil on the mountains; gravel road and compacted soil on the return trip

HIKING TIME: 2.5 hours

ACCESS: Open year-round, dawn–dusk

MAPS: Pamphlet available at visitor center and Marietta Welcome Center, phone (770) 429-1115; USGS Marietta

FACILITIES: Visitor center with restrooms at start and end of trail; a kind citizen provides dog water on return trip to visitor center.

IN BRIEF

This is the most challenging trail in this book and one of the most rewarding in the Atlanta area.

DESCRIPTION

On July 27, 1864, Union general William Sherman engaged Confederate forces under the command of General Joseph Johnston along a 5-mile front on the west side of Kennesaw Mountain, Little Kennesaw Mountain, Pigeon Hill, and Cheatham Hill. This battle marked the worst defeat of the Union Army during the Atlanta Campaign. Kennesaw Mountain National Battlefield commemorates the battle.

The first mile of the Burnt Hickory Loop is known as Kennesaw Mountain Trail and climbs 600 feet to the top of Big Kennesaw (the mountain's local name), following a combination of gravel roads and compacted-dirt paths. Keen eyes will spot Civil War–era entrenchments over the first 0.5 miles of the footpath. You'll also see a historic road, which crosscuts a modern gravel road at 0.3 miles. Rebel forces used this road to drag artillery to the mountaintop. For a scenic view at 0.5 miles, make the brief walk down an unmarked

UTM Trailhead Coordinates

UTM Zone (NAD27) 16S

Easting 0723730

Northing 3762652

Directions

Take I-75 to Exit 269, GA 5/Ernest Barrett Parkway. Turn left at the end of the ramp onto Barrett Parkway. Travel 1.9 miles and turn left on Old Highway 41. At 1.5 miles turn right on Stilesboro Road, then make an immediate left (0.1 mile) into Kennesaw National Battlefield Park (NBP). Walk toward a brown kiosk between the visitor center and Kennesaw Mountain Road.

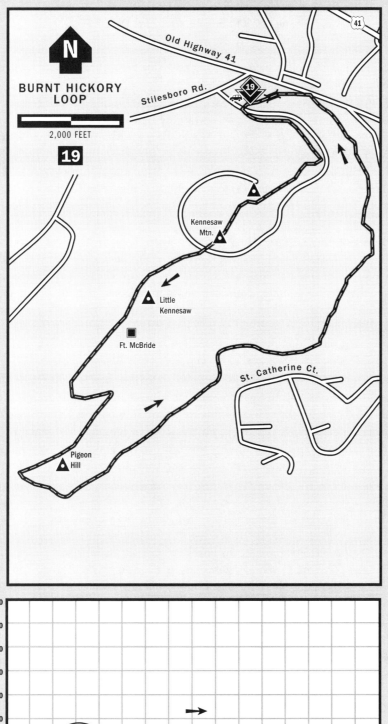

BURNT HICKORY LOOP

N

2,000 FEET

19

Old Highway 41

41

Stilesboro Rd.

19

Kennesaw
Mtn.

Little
Kennesaw

Ft. McBride

St. Catherine Ct.

Pigeon
Hill

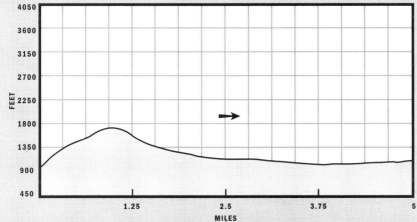

4050
3600
3150
2700
2250
1800
1350
900
450

FEET

1.25   2.5   3.75   5

MILES

path on the left. On clear days, the King and Queen and the Georgia Dome are visible from this vantage point.

The trail climbs a set of iron-railed concrete steps and turns left on a sidewalk. As you follow the sidewalk around to the right, the view to your left opens up for a good long-distance vista of Atlanta. It was from this site that Sherman first observed Atlanta, then home to a mere 10,000 residents. It had taken Sherman less than two months to move 60 miles from Ringgold to Marietta. But it would take more than two months to move the 12 miles from Marietta to Atlanta. While we were admiring the view, an American bald eagle skirted the mountain 40 feet below.

As you continue on the sidewalk, steps leave to the left; climb them to the massive Georgia Memorial. Dedicated on the 100th anniversary of the Battle of Kennesaw Mountain, the structure is a memorial to all Georgia-born generals who fought in that conflict. Continue straight ahead to the top of Kennesaw Mountain. Although this trail sees heavy use, there are many fewer hikers past the Georgia Memorial.

From the memorial, the footpath, which is initially paved, quickly returns to a rocky and root-strewn dirt trail as it passes Civil War–era cannon along the ridgelike mountaintop. The men stationed here saw the 100,000-man Union Army fill the valley beneath them as Sherman moved into position for a battle. At 0.9 miles the path breaks into full sun as it reaches the crest of Kennesaw Mountain, then begins a moderate-to-difficult descent to Kennesaw Mountain Road. Almost immediately, a side trail heads off to the left. Continue straight along the scenic ridge of Big Kennesaw. At 1 mile, the trail descends stairs to Mountain Road, which you can follow back to the visitor center for a total hike of 2 miles.

Across the road is a small parking lot and an interpretive sign telling the story of Little Kennesaw Mountain, which looms before and below the scenic overlook. The footpath descends a flight of concrete steps, joining a rocky dirt path at the bottom. The rocky nature of the path stunts tree growth, so you'll see massive post oaks and shortleaf pines that are only 30 feet tall. At 1.3 miles the trail reaches the gap between Big and Little Kennesaw and begins a moderate-to-difficult climb to the top of Little Kennesaw, alternating between sections of partial shade and full sun.

Four cannons that occupy the top of Little Kennesaw (1.5 miles) at Civil War–era Fort McBride mark the start of the most difficult portion of the trail. The National Park Service has repeatedly reworked the steep-sided and rock-strewn trail in this area to make it easier to navigate, with limited success. In 2005 the trail was reworked and remarked, with only a few switchbacks. A pine blowdown at 2.1 miles marks the gap between Little Kennesaw and Pigeon Hill.

Massive boulders atop extended sheets of granite mark the top of Pigeon Hill, the only area on Burnt Hickory Loop that saw extensive fighting during the Battle of Kennesaw Mountain. Union troops were repulsed before reaching the top of the mountain. The hill drew its name from the passenger pigeon, a now-extinct bird that once nested here, blackening the skies during migrations. At 2.3 miles, turn left at a brown sign that says simply "East." This marks the return trail to the visitor center.

Descending gently over the next 0.3 miles, the trail swings to the left and joins a gravel road at a signed intersection. Turn left and follow the relatively level gravel road through a second-growth hardwood forest punctuated with loblolly pine and native magnolia (Southern grandifolia). At 3.4 miles you'll see houses off to the right; a few steps farther on, you'll find a wooden fence to prevent you from accidentally walking into somebody's backyard. Along this fence, a caring citizen leaves a plastic bucket with water for animals.

After the fence ends at 3.6 miles, the gravel road continues to the marked Kennesaw Mountain Civilian Conservation Corps (CCC) campsite off to the left, just past a gravel road that heads off to the left. The men who lived at this camp made many of the initial improvements to the park and discovered the grave of the unknown soldier at Cheatham Hill (see Cheatham Hill Trail). A few steps past the level campsite are the remains of the headquarters building. Almost nothing remains of the CCC camp, whose modular buildings were transported to house workers elsewhere.

Leaving the gravel road at 4.3 miles, the trail bears left, then turns right at a map stand 0.1 mile ahead, continuing past a blowdown courtesy of the southern pine beetle. As traffic noise increases, the trail bears left, entering full sun in an open field at 4.7 miles. The traffic light to the entrance of Kennesaw Mountain NBP is off to the right, and the visitor center comes into view shortly as the trail slowly curves left alongside an open field. Just before the visitor center, you'll see the Georgia Monument on the left, across the paved Mountain Road.

NEARBY ATTRACTIONS

Marietta offers some of the best antiques shopping in the state around the antebellum square 1 mile east of the visitor center. Adjacent to the historic depot downtown are the Marietta History Museum and Scarlett on the Square, a *Gone with the Wind* movie museum.

20 KOLB'S FARM LOOP

KEY AT-A-GLANCE INFORMATION

LENGTH: 5.5 miles

CONFIGURATION: Loop

DIFFICULTY: Moderate

SCENERY: Portions of a Civil War battlefield, some good creek views

EXPOSURE: Alternating full sun and shade on the west side, mostly full shade on the east side

TRAFFIC: Heavy

TRAIL SURFACE: Compact soil; some of the hike is on gravel roads

HIKING TIME: 3 hours

ACCESS: Open year-round, dawn–dusk

MAPS: Available at Kennesaw Mountain National Battlefield Park visitor center; USGS Marietta

FACILITIES: Water on trail near Kolb's Farm

SPECIAL COMMENTS: Kennesaw Mountain National Battlefield Park was Georgia's first Important Birding Area (IBA). Horses are allowed on portions of the trail.

UTM Trailhead Coordinates

UTM Zone (NAD27) 16S

Easting   0721431

Northing   3757039

IN BRIEF

The trail explores the north end of a Civil War battlefield. It is also designed to attract birds, from common yellow finches to the stunning scarlet tanager.

DESCRIPTION

Kennesaw Mountain National Battlefield Park was the first area in Georgia to be designated an important bird area (IBA). Migratory birds use the park extensively during the fall and spring, as do year-round species. Among the birds you may spot along the trail are warblers, thrushes, and tanagers. Larger birds include orioles, rails, and hawks.

Turn right on a gravel road, passing around a brown gate that excludes vehicular traffic, and immediately begin a short, moderate climb to the trail's high point, a ridge some 30 feet above and 600 feet behind the parking lot. On the east side of this ridge, on July 27, 1864, about 8,000 Union troops under the

----

Directions ⟶

Take I-75 North to Exit 263, South Marietta Parkway/120 Loop/Southern Poly. At the end of the ramp, turn right toward Southern Poly and the Cobb Civic Center. Cross Franklin Road at 0.1 mile and Cobb Parkway (US 41) at 0.5 miles. At 2.6 miles the 120 Loop curves left, crosses Atlanta Street, and passes under some railroad tracks. Less than 0.1 mile later, immediately after the tracks, turn left on Powder Springs Road and follow it 3.9 miles to Cheatham Hill Road. Turn right and travel 1.6 miles to the Kolb's Farm Trail parking lot on the left. Use the second driveway to enter it. After parking, walk to the south end of the lot over a compacted-soil trail to reach a large rock in a gravel road: this marks the start and end of Kolb's Farm Loop.

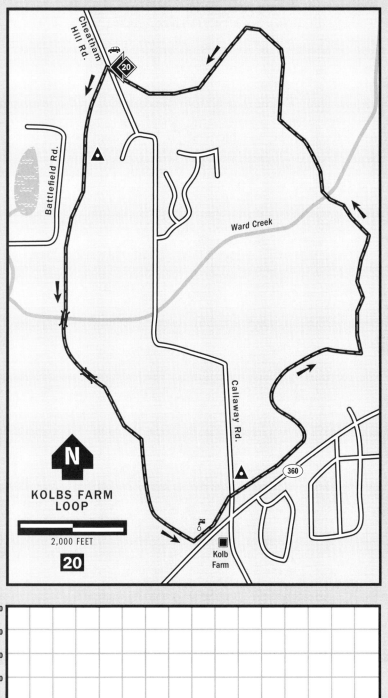

KOLBS FARM LOOP

2,000 FEET

20

Cheatham Hill Rd.

Battlefield Rd.

Ward Creek

Callaway Rd.

360

Kolb Farm

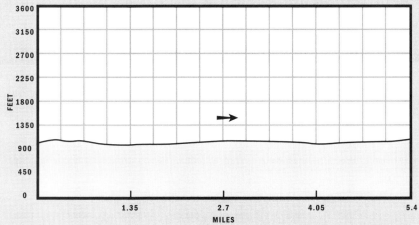

command of General George Thomas began to assemble for a frontal assault on a heavily fortified Confederate line at Cheatham Hill (see hike 16, page 80), about 0.4 miles due east of this spot. The ensuing battle was the Union Army's worst defeat during the Atlanta Campaign.

The trail levels and begins to descend through a second-growth forest mostly composed of red maple and a number of varieties of pine, with native dogwood, especially alongside the road. At 0.8 miles the trail begins a moderate-to-difficult descent to John Ward Creek as the forest becomes mostly pine, including a number of tall, ramrod-straight loblollies. About halfway down the hill is the first cleared field, designed to attract birds. It is not unusual to see at least a couple of birders on the west side of the loop trail.

As it approaches the creek, Kolb's Farm Loop begins to level off and a gravel road heads off to the right at just under 1 mile. This road is a walk-around for horses, which would destroy the wooden-planked boardwalk ahead. About 0.1 mile later, the pathway becomes a boardwalk a few inches above a marshy area surrounding John Ward Creek. After crossing the creek and more marshland, the boardwalk ends and the gravel horse path returns. The smell of honeysuckle wafts through the air, and you can see homes off to the right.

Approaching 1.2 miles the trail in this area has been reworked, so mind the markings and continue on the new trail, straight ahead, skirting the end of a field. As the trail curves right, there is a large stand of bamboo on the right. Returning to the forest at 1.5 miles, the loop trail begins a 0.3-mile climb. At the peak of this hill, Kolb's Farm Trail slowly curves right, and the sound of traffic noise grows louder, continuing for the next mile as the pathway parallels Powder Springs Road.

Undergrowth increases and Virginia creeper and wild grape abound. A working water fountain on the right side of the path at 2.4 miles is ready to quench the thirst of hikers and dogs. Immediately after passing the water fountain, you can see the road and a development across the street. These homes were built on the site of major fighting in the Battle of Kolb's Farm. A few steps farther on is the first view of Kolb's Farm.

Peter Valentine Kolb came to Cobb County in the 1830s and built this dog-trot cabin composed of an open center hall with four rooms, two on either side. Kolb was wealthy compared to others in the area—he had enough money to build four fireplaces. Sometime after 1845 he enclosed the dogtrot, now an open center hall. In the early 1960s, the National Park Service restored the cabin to its appearance at the time of the Battle of Kennesaw Mountain. At this point the loop trail begins to skirt the northern edge of the battlefield.

After a gravel road heads off to the right, the pathway reaches Cheatham Hill Road. Turn right at the paved road and cross Powder Springs Road at the traffic light. Continue to a small parking lot just east of Kolb's Farm. There are historic markers describing the house and the battle, in addition to a small family cemetery. Do not approach the house, which is a private residence.

Return to the light, cross Callaway Road, and then turn left. Cross Powder Springs Road, continue north from the road, and turn right onto a walkway with stone walls that leads to an open field. The path roughly parallels an entrenchment held by Union troops during the battle. These men fired on Confederate general Hood's right flank as Hood attacked the Union's Army of the Ohio under the command of General John Schofield on June 22, 1864. Historic markers on the right side of the trail use maps to tell the story of the battle in depth.

Turning left at 2.7 miles, the trail becomes forested and reenters heavy shade. Signs indicate the trail goes to the visitor center and Cheatham Hill, guiding hikers to make the turn. After reaching the top of a ridge at 2.9 miles, the trail begins an extended moderate descent to John Ward Creek. You'll see houses on the left 0.2 miles later, then enter a steep-sided ravine with large trees.

After the loop trail narrows and goes around a large granite boulder, it becomes heavily rooted and rocky. To cross a ravine, Kolb's Farm Loop makes a short, steep descent to a stone-and-dirt bridge, then quickly ascends before continuing to John Ward Creek.

The pathway turns to gravel roadbed at 3.5 miles, and you'll occasionally see houses on the right. The final descent to John Ward Creek traverses a valley. At 3.9 miles the trail splits. On the left the footpath climbs a low ridge and parallels the second trail, which runs adjacent to the river. If the river is running high, the trail to the right will be blocked. After 0.2 miles the trails rejoin on the ridge. If you took the trail to the right, turn right at the three-way intersection.

At John Ward Creek, there are two bridges about 100 feet apart to take you across. After the second bridge, a trail enters from the right. Over the next 0.5 miles there are four Y-intersections. Always take the trail to the left as you follow a wide, roadlike path. At 4.8 miles, cross an earthwork that was held by Maney's Brigade during the Battle of Kennesaw Mountain. Turn left when the trail reaches a T-intersection 0.2 miles later. From this point on, there are a number of side trails on the right to Cheatham Hill. After crossing a stone bridge at 5.1 miles, the trail begins the ascent to the Kolb's Farm Loop parking area, curving left and then bearing right as it leaves the roadbed 500 feet after the bridge. The final moderate ascent brings you to Cheatham Hill Road. Cross the street and turn right to return to your car.

NEARBY ATTRACTIONS

The Kennesaw Mountain National Battlefield Park has a museum discussing the battles fought in or near what is now the park, in addition to describing the entire Atlanta Campaign. It is open daily from 8:30 a.m. to 5 p.m., except on Thanksgiving and Christmas.

21   NEW ECHOTA TRAIL

KEY AT-A-GLANCE INFORMATION

LENGTH: 1.9 miles
CONFIGURATION: Loop
DIFFICULTY: Easy
SCENERY: Cherokee capital, forested wetlands, overhead view of creek
EXPOSURE: Full sun, except on the woods section of the hike
TRAFFIC: Light
TRAIL SURFACE: Compact soil
HIKING TIME: 2 hours
ACCESS: Tuesday–Saturday, 9 a.m.–5 p.m.; Sunday, 2–5:30 p.m. Closed Mondays (except holidays) and on Thanksgiving, December 25, and January 1. Closed Tuesday when open Monday.
MAPS: Available inside visitor center; USGS Calhoun North
FACILITIES: Restrooms, picnic tables
SPECIAL COMMENTS: New Echota was the only capital of the Cherokee Nation in the eastern United States.

IN BRIEF

This hike explores the site of a Cherokee city built as its seat of government in 1825, then climbs a ridge along a creek that was a popular campsite when the national council was in session.

DESCRIPTION

The hopes and dreams of the Cherokee Nation rested on New Echota, the city that became their capital during a nationalistic movement in the mid-1820s. Today the once-busy streets are quiet, a chilling testament to the greed of humankind.

In about 1400, moving west into what would become the State of Georgia, the Cherokee claimed the land from north Georgia to the Ohio River Valley and west to the Mississippi. Over a period of slightly more than 100 years, England and later the United States repeatedly encroached on the Cherokee's "Enchanted Land." In 1832 the State of Georgia delivered a major blow to the Cherokee Nation's dreams—they gave it away to European settlers in a lottery. There was a major problem: Georgia did not own the land at the time. Three years later a small group of Cherokee (fewer than 500 out of 16,000 signed the corrupt Treaty of New Echota, ceding the land

UTM Trailhead Coordinates

UTM Zone (NAD27) 16S

Easting   0691808

Northing   3823869

Directions

Take I-75 North to Exit 317, GA 225/Joseph Vann Highway. Turn right at the end of the ramp and travel 0.7 miles to the entrance to New Echota State Park. Turn right and follow the road around to the right. Park and walk to the entrance to the visitor center, near the west end of the lot.

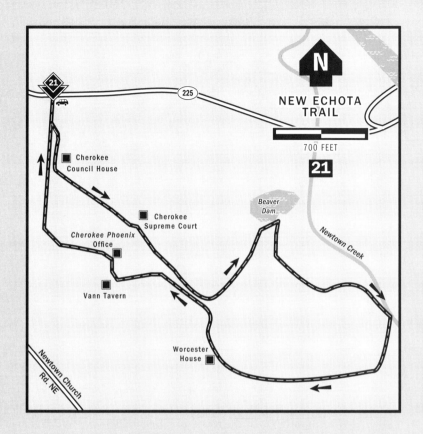

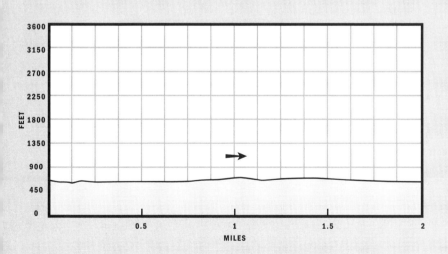

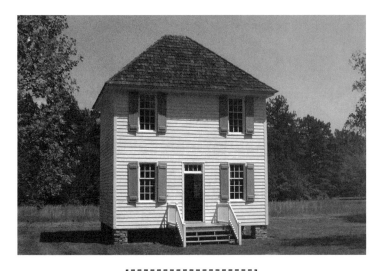

Cherokee Supreme Court

to the state. Under pressure from Andrew Jackson, the Senate approved the treaty by a single vote, and the stage was set for one of the greatest tragedies in American history, the Trail of Tears.

As the Cherokee left, settlers moved in and used the homes they had left behind. One building became a schoolhouse, another a general store. Other homes were simply left to rot. In 1952 the land was put up for sale, and local residents, aware of the historic importance of the town, purchased 200 acres and donated it to the state, which began an excavation of the city, identifying the sites of many original buildings' foundations. Only Samuel Worcester's home remained intact. Worcester, the white missionary the Cherokee called "the Messenger," was a pivotal figure in the legal battle waged in the U.S. Supreme Court. In *Worcester v. Georgia,* the court held that the state could not extend its laws upon the Cherokee Nation. Both Georgia and the federal government chose to ignore the ruling.

After paying an entrance fee of $4 per person and visiting the small but exquisite museum, leave the visitor center and turn right. The hike begins in a middle-class Cherokee homestead, re-created from buildings taken from across north Georgia. The homes of the Cherokee were virtually indistinguishable from the homes of settlers in the late 1820s. The Cherokee used many of the same technologies the settlers did, from spinning yarn to farming with plowshares. In the farm re-created here, there is a home, barn, smokehouse, and corncrib. Exit behind the home onto a dirt street and walk toward the town proper. The next building on the tour of the town is the Cherokee Council House. This two-story building housed a bicameral council similar in many ways to the U.S. House and Senate. It was here that laws were proposed and enacted for the entire Cherokee Nation.

After exiting the Council House, turn right and walk to the Cherokee Supreme Court, a white building on stone footers. Cherokee law was argued here, just as

U.S. law is in the Supreme Court. As you leave the building, turn left and walk toward the common Cherokee house. John Rodgers, a "countryman" (a white man with a Cherokee wife), lived on this site. The original home is gone, but a representative cabin was brought in from the hills nearby. Rodgers was not the only white man living in the village with the Cherokee. John Wheeler, a printer for the *Cherokee Phoenix*, married the sister of Elias Boudinot and lived in the town, as did Daniel McCoy, who ran the only year-round general store there.

As you leave the farmhouse, look for a dirt road entering the forest. Turn left and walk down it. As the road begins to curve right, you'll see Newtown Trail on the left at 0.4 miles. Step down, then rock-hop over a tiny rivulet to reach the footpath. Follow the wide trail as it bears left through a floodplain after a side path heads off to the right. The interpreted hike identifies the flora and fauna of the area and explains their significance in everyday Cherokee life. The sweetgum tree (identified early in the hike) was of great importance to the Cherokee and grew well in this wet environment. Not only did the tree provide a kind of chewing gum, it also had medicinal properties and was applied to wounds.

Watch for the water oak, sometimes called a possum oak, and its single rounded leaf. Its smaller acorn, which features a flattened cap, is popular with many of the animals that inhabit or use the area near the river. Another tree in this diverse hardwood forest is the shagbark hickory, used by both the Cherokee and settlers to smoke meat because of the sweet flavor its smoke imparted.

The trail dips to a pond created by an active beaver dam. A dock off the trail to the left allows visitors a good look into the pond's clear water. Return to Newtown Trail, where you'll pass through a blowdown created by the southern pine beetle. As the trail reenters hardwood forest, it curves right and begins a short climb to a low ridge joining Newtown Creek at 0.9 miles. A few steps farther along you'll reach an overlook deck with a picturesque view of the creek that flows in from the right, turns until it runs almost directly at the overlook, then turns again as it runs into a solid rock wall beneath the overlook. Less than 0.25 miles later it joins the Oostanaula River, which eventually ends up in the Gulf of Mexico.

One of the more interesting interpretive signs points out a dramatic change in the trail's fauna caused by the hardwood forest quickly changing to a new-growth pine forest. Until the late 1940s, the field was cultivated as part of a farm. When the field went fallow, fast-growing pine quickly took over. Slower-growing hardwoods will take time to supplant them. The trail curves right, coming to the Worcester house at 1.3 miles. From the home, turn right on the gravel road in front of the house and follow it around to Vann's Tavern. Named for James Vann, a wily, intemperate mixed-blood Cherokee, the tavern was moved from Vann's Ferry, which crossed the Chattahoochee River and was the major entry point to the Cherokee Nation. There was a walk-up window at the tavern, where travelers could buy a drink before continuing on their journey.

From the tavern, walk to the office of the *Cherokee Phoenix*, the first newspaper published by Native Americans. From 1828 until the Cherokee Nation ran out of money in 1833 (the federal government began to withhold payments agreed to in treaties), the paper was the legal organ of the Nation. The cellar of the home of Elias Boudinot, the first publisher of the paper, is adjacent to the building. Follow the road in front of the Phoenix and Boudinot's cellar to the right, and turn right at the dirt road just past the trees. This returns you to the parking area.

NEARBY ATTRACTIONS

Further explore the life of the Cherokee in north Georgia at James Vann's home. Built in the early 1800s, the home reflects an opulent lifestyle not normally attributed to the Cherokee. Vann was one of the richest men in the Southeast when this house was completed. Turn right out of New Echota State Park and continue 17.6 miles. The home and a museum are on the left just after Alternate 52. Open Tuesday through Saturday, 9 a.m.–5 p.m.; Sunday, 2 p.m.–5:30 p.m.; $4 per person.

PICKETT'S MILL TRAIL

IN BRIEF

This trail explores the site of a decisive Confederate victory during the Atlanta Campaign, then takes hikers down the path Union soldiers trod as they advanced down a valley toward the Confederate Army's right flank.

DESCRIPTION

The Battle of Pickett's Mill was a mistake. Sherman had hit on a successful plan—engage the enemy while outflanking them—and tried to duplicate it here in the rolling hills south of Kingston, Georgia. Union troops had engaged the Confederates at New Hope Church, west of Pickett's Mill. Sherman ordered General George Thomas to find the left end of the Rebel line and outflank Confederate general

----

Directions

Take I-75 North to Exit 277, GA 92. At the end of the ramp, turn left and immediately get in the right-hand lane. Drive 0.2 miles to the traffic line, then turn right on Lake Acworth Drive and follow it 3.7 miles to Cobb Parkway. Turn right and move into the left-hand lane. Continue 1.5 miles then turn left on Dallas-Acworth Highway. At 4.1 miles turn left at a four-way stop on Cedarcrest Road (GA 92 South). Two miles later, you'll see the Pickett's Mill Battlefield family shelter on the right, but do not turn here. Turn right on Due West Road at 2.6 miles, then drive 1.8 miles and make a left on Mt. Tabor Church Road. Travel 0.4 miles to Pickett's Mill Historic Site. Turn right and go through a wooden gate. The visitor center is 0.6 miles down the road, on the left. Park, then walk to the entrance of the blue wood-and-stone visitor center. After paying the $3 admission, exit the other side of the building and follow a concrete path to a wooden-deck overlook. This is the trailhead.

KEY AT-A-GLANCE INFORMATION

LENGTH: 3.1 miles

CONFIGURATION: Loop

DIFFICULTY: Moderate

SCENERY: Multiple creekside settings with cascades

EXPOSURE: Most of the trail in full shade

TRAFFIC: Moderate

TRAIL SURFACE: Compact soil; gravel and historic roads

HIKING TIME: 2 hours

ACCESS: Open year-round; closed Monday, except legal holidays

MAPS: Map with marker descriptions and troop movements available for purchase at visitor center; USGS Dallas

FACILITIES: Visitor center with bathrooms and a small museum; picnic tables

SPECIAL COMMENTS: Excellent DVD presentation on the battle of Pickett's Mill

- -

UTM Trailhead Coordinates

UTM Zone (NAD27) 16S

Easting   0707016

Northing 3761318

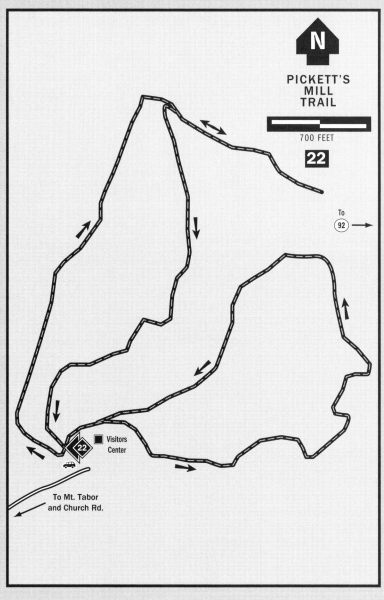

N

PICKETT'S MILL TRAIL

700 FEET

22

To 92 →

Visitors Center

22

To Mt. Tabor and Church Rd.

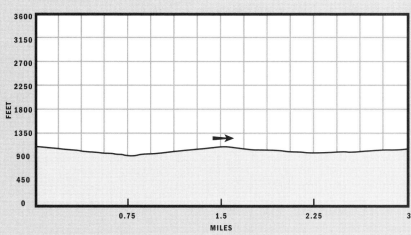

Joseph Johnston once again. Thomas and a subordinate, General O. O. Howard, mistook a salient in the Rebel line for the end of the line and ordered an attack—against the best tactical commander in the Western theater of operations, Patrick Cleburne. Cleburne once defeated Sherman himself, although Sherman had outnumbered Cleburne ten to one at the time.

Advancing under fire down a valley on May 27, 1864, Union soldiers were trapped by Cleburne's men. Some Yankees did take higher ground, eventually continuing the advance, but they, too, were forced back. A second wave of Union soldiers, intended to reinforce the first, ended up to the east of the main attack. After withstanding heavy losses, the Union soldiers retreated under cover of darkness. The loss was such a stinging blow to Sherman that he did not mention it in his memoirs.

Pickett's Mill contains three separate trails (red, white, and blue), covering each of the historically important sites within the 765-acre park. This narrative combines the three trails into one hike. From the overlook, follow the red-blazed trail to the right. Quickly joining a gravel road, the trail descends through a mostly pine forest punctuated by an occasional red maple. After 0.1 mile the red trail turns right. Before the turn, just below you to the left, is the area of heaviest fighting. Here Confederates repelled three Yankee attacks, but there was no time for the Rebels to build a trench line.

After turning right, the red trail descends through a pine forest. Burn markings on the bottom of the trees have nothing to do with the Civil War but tell the story of a more recent forest fire. Throughout the park, you can see entrenchments near each of the developed trails. The first one is on the right at 0.2 miles. A cornfield on the left at 0.3 miles marks the farthest Union penetration during the Battle of Pickett's Mill. At this point the road curves left into the cornfield and ends, but the pathway continues, entering a pine forest on the right side of the road. Less than 0.1 mile later, the trail makes a sharp left and descends to a bridge over a dry creek, then turns rocky as it climbs to a low ridge through a forest of red maple, American beech, and native dogwood.

Just less than 1 mile into the hike, the blue trail rejoins the red trail, and the red trail turns right. Turn left on the blue trail and continue an extended climb over the next 0.6 miles. Near the trail at 1 mile are the rifle pits that the Confederate cavalry quickly dug in an attempt to delay a secondary Union attack. The delay tactic worked—a combined force of Confederate infantry and cavalry had time to establish a line some 500 feet to the rear. As the trail climbs, it again passes through territory Union soldiers held for some of the battle, then rejoins the red trail and continues past the overlook at the trailhead.

Now on the white trail, the path curves to the right just past the visitor center. A few feet after the center and to the right in a mostly pine forest is a historic road. Off to the left are additional entrenchments. The gravel road continues downhill but gradually levels off, coming to a side trail at 1.7 miles that rejoins the main trail 0.2 miles later. Reaching a Y-intersection at 2 miles, take the path to the left. Less than 100 feet on, the path makes a sharp right, entering the forest and leaving the gravel road at an "Area Closed" sign. The path briefly descends to the site of a federal artillery emplacement.

Turn around and retrace your steps to the Y-intersection. Turn left and follow the mostly level path 0.1 mile, where the white trail heads off to the right. Continue straight, making an easy descent to a road on the left. Turn left, although the road does continue straight. Now descending much more steeply, the trail enters Little Pumpkinvine Creek Valley, so called because the winding river resembles a pumpkin vine when viewed from above. The Georgia legislature officially renamed the stream Pickett's Mill Creek in the 1990s.

In this area, the Union assault formed late in the afternoon on May 27, 1864. Take a few minutes to enjoy the now serene surroundings. Retrace your steps to the top of the hill and turn left on the combined red, white, and blue trails, where the trail enters "the Ravine." The next 0.5 miles of the trail takes hikers along the path that Union soldiers used to advance on Confederate positions in the vicinity of the visitor center. A relatively small number of Rebels, entrenched at the tops of the hills on either side, poured deadly fire on the advancing Yankees. Union commanders, who had charged the Confederate line three times, decided to dig in and hold their positions. Supporting drives did not weaken the Confederate line, and under cover of darkness the Yankees retreated.

As you leave the valley, the trailhead is directly in front of you.

POOLES MILL COVERED BRIDGE

IN BRIEF

This trail meanders down a ridge to Pooles Mill Covered Bridge and explores Settindown Creek, the river the bridge spans. The cascading falls after the bridge on the left are a great place to enjoy the river.

DESCRIPTION

A Cherokee trading path ran about 1 mile north of Pooles Mill. In 1804, under terms laid out in the Treaty of Tellico, this path became the federal highway that connected Savannah to Nashville. By the time the Cherokee chief George Welch established the first mill on the site in 1820, traffic was steadily increasing on the road. Welch sided with the Cherokees, advocating removal in 1835 rather than fighting the settlers who had already stolen the Cherokees' land. He left Georgia soon after signing the supplement to the Treaty of New Echota on March 1, 1836. According to the Historical Society of Forsyth County, the federal government reimbursed Welch $719.50 for the gristmill.

Jacob Scudder was an entrepreneur with a number of businesses in a town known as Scudders near the intersection of Matt Highway and Old Federal Road, north of Pooles Mill. Today, little remains of the small town, but it was Scudder, a white man, who took over Chief Welch's mill. Scudder, who married Welch's sister-in-law, purchased the land from

KEY AT-A-GLANCE INFORMATION

LENGTH: 1.1 miles

CONFIGURATION: Out-and-back

DIFFICULTY: Easy

SCENERY: Covered bridge; falls and cascades along Settindown Creek

EXPOSURE: Full sun

TRAFFIC: Moderate

TRAIL SURFACE: Compact soil and paved roadbed

HIKING TIME: 1 hour

ACCESS: Open year-round, dawn–dusk

MAPS: USGS Matt

FACILITIES: Restrooms, picnic tables with grills, pavilion that can be rented from Forsyth County, children's playground

SPECIAL COMMENTS: Pooles Mill is one of 12 covered bridges in Georgia.

UTM Trailhead Coordinates

UTM Zone (NAD27) 16S

Easting   0753866

Northing   3797452

Directions

From GA 400 turn left on GA 369, at the first traffic light after the controlled access portion of the road ends. Travel 10.1 miles to Pooles Mill Road and turn left. Pooles Mill parking area is 0.7 miles down on the right.

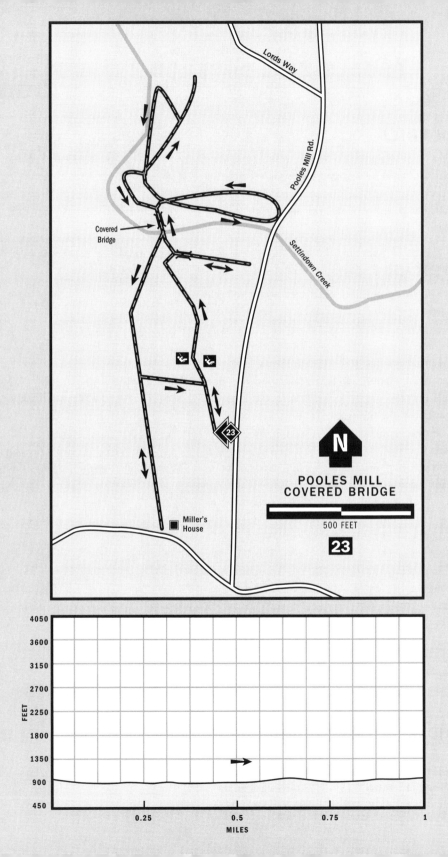

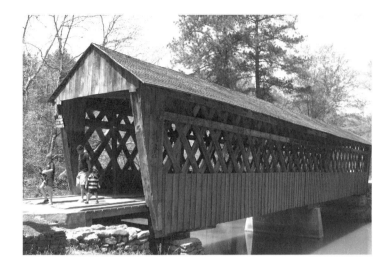

Pooles Mill covered bridge

the man who won it during the Sixth Georgia Land Lottery. He added a sawmill to the existing gristmill, and, shortly before he died, transferred the title to his sons, who sold it to Dr. D. L. Pool. It is not known why landmarks bearing Pool's name are spelled with an "e." By the time the mill ceased operations in 1947, electricity had replaced water as the power source of choice, and chickens had replaced grain and cotton. The mill was burned down by vandals in 1959.

Since the Old Federal Highway was north of the mill, Pooles Mill Bridge began as a simple wooden structure to span Settindown Creek between the mill and the main road. In 1899 the bridge was washed away, and the county contracted a millwright to build a new bridge. He quit before completing the bridge, and Bud Gentry was hired. Gentry is generally credited with building the bridge.

From the trailhead kiosk at the north end of the parking lot, the compacted-dirt trail meanders through a children's playground with swings and slides. At the top of the knoll, a "trail tree" marked the way to the bridge before the county opened the park in 1997. A pavilion to the right of the trail contains the park's restrooms.

From the knoll, the trail splits—one side goes directly to the bridge, the other to a small garden area maintained by the county. Just before the bridge, the trails rejoin, and asphalt-paved roads enter from both the left and the right. Turn right and walk along Settindown Creek to reach the modern bridge over the creek. There are good places to photograph the covered bridge from along the bank, especially as sunset approaches. Picnic tables line the creek.

Return to the bridge at 0.3 miles and cross it, then turn right and follow the road on the other side, as far as the modern bridge. From this side you can exit the park and carefully walk to the center of the modern bridge for an excellent view of the covered bridge. Be extremely careful with young children, though, because drivers frequently speed here. Return to the bridge and turn left on the original roadway connecting Pooles Mill to the Old Federal Highway. To get an idea of what roads were like before the modern, paved road became popular in the 1920s, follow this rough road down to the chain-link fence that marks private property at 0.6 miles.

Turn around and watch for a well-worn path heading off to the right about halfway back to the bridge. Turn right and follow it over two sets of rock outcrops down to the bottom of a set of cascading falls typical of north Georgia. A chain-link fence prevents visitors from following the riverbank to the right, but turn left and begin climbing a series of rocks as the water shoots through, around, and over the rocks in the river. Just below the top of the rock, watch for metal spikes driven into the granite, as if to anchor a structure.

Return to the bridge and cross it, but instead of following the trail back, continue straight ahead on the paved road as it rises to the modern street. Across the street on the left is the house where the miller lived. Mills in north Georgia were often operated by a man other than the owner, and part of the miller's compensation was a home. This house is privately owned; do not approach it. Return down the path to a crossover trail on the left, just before the playground, and take it to return to your car.

NEARBY ATTRACTIONS

From early to mid-October, the Cumming Country Fair and Festival offers a look back at Cherokee history; exhibits include a seven-sided council house. Blackburn's Tavern, one of the town's few remaining buildings, has been restored and now sits in this area. A covered bridge has been added in recent years to permit access to this area. Additional displays at the fair include an extensive collection of pre-1930 steam-powered building equipment , two working mills, a blacksmith shop, and a 1940s-era cotton gin. We particularly enjoyed the working sawmill, which demonstrates how the sawmill at Pooles Mill would have worked. Be sure to spend a few minutes at the quilting bee.

SILVER COMET TRAIL: ROCKMART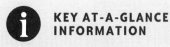

IN BRIEF

Silver Comet Trail in Rockmart follows the Seaboard Line tracks, now a concrete trail, to the old slate quarry and into downtown Rockmart. More than 100 years old, the city offers a delightful break, whether you stop for lunch or just to window shop.

DESCRIPTION

Unlike Silver Comet Trail between Mavell Road and Floyd Road (see pages 66 and 113), or near Pumpkinvine Trestle at the end of Wild Horse Creek Trail (see page 29), the trail in the vicinity of Rockmart is only lightly used. The railroad bed in Rockmart is significantly older than that near Mavell Road. Seaboard needed a railroad from Atlanta to Alabama. Rather than build the route themselves, they purchased an existing line from Alabama to Cartersville, Georgia, and built the additional track from Rockmart to Atlanta in 1904. Coot's Lake Beach, for which the trailhead is named, is a pay-per-use facility adjacent to the trailhead.

Walk to the front of the parking lot and turn right. A short access trail makes a short drop to the Silver Comet. Turn left on the wide, concrete-paved path and almost immediately cross Coot's Lake Road at an intersection with no traffic light. After the intersection, the Silver

KEY AT-A-GLANCE INFORMATION

LENGTH: 9.5 miles

CONFIGURATION: Out-and-back

DIFFICULTY: Easy

SCENERY: 2 large creeks in the city of Rockmart, railroads, slate quarry

EXPOSURE: Full sun

TRAFFIC: Light

TRAIL SURFACE: Concrete

HIKING TIME: 4 hours

ACCESS: Open year-round, dawn–dusk

MAPS: Available for a fee at Silver Comet Express (Floyd Road); USGS Rockmart South, Rockmart North

FACILITIES: Port-a-john at parking lot, restrooms in Rockmart City Hall

SPECIAL COMMENTS: There are few hikers on Silver Comet Trail outside Cobb County. There are many things for kids to see and do around Rockmart, making this a great family hike.

Directions

Take I-75 to Exit 288, Main Street/GA 113. At the stop sign, turn left and go 2.6 miles to where the road bears left at a marked intersection and becomes Etowah Drive. Travel 0.3 miles, then make a right on GA 113, Airport Road. Take Airport 18.3 miles to US 278. Turn left and travel 2.7 miles to Coot's Lake Road. Turn left, and travel 0.1 mile to the entrance to the parking lot on the right.

UTM Trailhead Coordinates

UTM Zone (NAD27) 16S

Easting   0684369

Northing   3761200

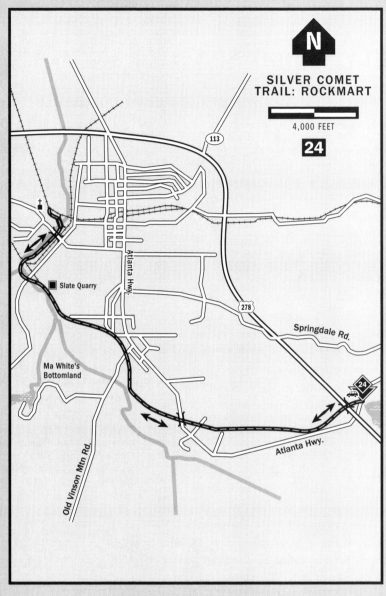

**SILVER COMET
TRAIL: ROCKMART**

4,000 FEET

24

113

Atlanta Hwy.

278

Springdale Rd.

Slate Quarry

Ma White's
Bottomland

24

Atlanta Hwy.

Old Vinson Mtn Rd.

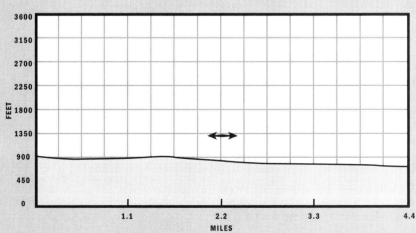

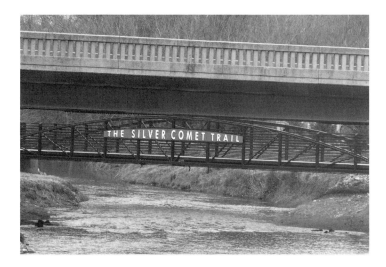

Bridge over Euharlee Creek

Comet curves to the right, leaving the original roadbed of the Seaboard Line, then curves back to the left as it begins a fairly sharp descent to a narrow, unlit underpass. As the trail exits the underpass, it begins an equally steep rise and returns to the original roadbed. You'll notice various mature pines near the trail as the path imperceptibly descends almost the entire distance to downtown Rockmart.

Watch down the hill on the left for an old shed at 0.3 miles. Sheds like these were common throughout north Georgia and the Blue Ridge Mountains before the 20th century. The shed is a good example of form following geography. Because mountain fields were frequently far apart, farmers would build a small shed for each field, rather than storing all the equipment in a single barn. On the right, past the shed, are sharp cliffs exposing the red Georgia clay in a man-made cut. At mile marker 34, the trail gently curves right. The Silver Comet's raised roadbed after the curve is made of the debris that was removed to create the railroad cut. At 0.9 miles the trail crosses McDowell Road, a two-lane dirt road.

Another cut begins at 1.5 miles, where the roadbed has been dug out of the mountain. Work has recently been done in this area because of a spate of tropical storms that raked Georgia in fall 2004. At 1.8 miles the trail passes under the Atlanta Highway; after this, you'll see additional cliffs that were created when the railroad was built. The trail slowly curves right, passing a small, clear pond on the left and crossing Vinson Mountain Road on a trestle. In the middle of the trestle, look left and you can see the entrance to the Van Wert parking lot.

Van Wert, originally the seat of Paulding County, is pretty much a forgotten town. When Polk County split off in 1851, Dallas became Paulding's county seat, and Cedartown became Polk's county seat, leaving Van Wert to struggle without the additional revenue generated by being a government center. In 1872 Seaborn Jones sealed the fate of struggling Van Wert when he donated land to form the village of Rockmart. The railroad built a depot in Rockmart and bypassed Van Wert.

Just past the trestle, the Van Wert parking area access trail heads off to the right, quickly descending to the parking lot. The Silver Comet begins a long, gradual curve to the left as the area known as White Bottom opens up on the left. A sign on the trail identifies the area as Ma White's bottomland, a shorter version of the original name. The Whites owned most of the land, and when her husband died, Ma White continued to run the farm.

The Silver Comet begins a sweeping curve to the right as it joins Thompson Creek, which you will see at 3.5 miles. From this point on through the city of Rockmart, the trail runs near this creek or the larger Euharlee Creek. Notice that the creek is running through a gorge carved from slate on your left. Rockmart Slate Quarry, complete with a railroad siding, is ahead on the right. One of the reasons the railroad ran to Rockmart was because it could generate income hauling slate from this quarry. Formed some 600 million years ago, a vast ancient sea deposited layers of sediments that, over time, became slate. A popular roofing material until the 1920s, slate was replaced by asbestos shingles. By that time a new use had been developed for the rock—it was used as an aggregate to strengthen cement.

At 3.8 miles the trail appears to rise to a road. But just before you begin the climb, a second paved trail heads off to the left, traveling under Hutchings Mountain Road. After the underpass, which the Silver Comet shares with nearby Simpson Creek, the landscape opens into a wide, level plain populated by massive oak trees. Continuing on the left, Simpson Creek runs alongside the trail to its confluence with the lyrically named Euharlee Creek. Shortly after the confluence, Silver Comet Trail curves abruptly to the right, passing under other tracks also owned by CSX. On the right, after an easy climb, you'll see a cotton gin at Beauregard Street, where the trail becomes the Rockmart Riverwalk, lined with black lampposts.

Passing under Church Street, the Silver Comet enters downtown Rockmart. In recent years this town has undergone a remarkable transformation, in part thanks to the increasing use of Silver Comet Trail. Upscale shopping and new restaurants join a century-old church and a police station. A wooden bridge crosses Euharlee Creek, allowing hikers access to Seaborn Jones Park. Dedicated in 2002, the park is a great addition to Silver Comet Trail, with picnic tables and large open areas. Turn right and continue to the bridge over Euharlee Creek to take the Silver Comet north out of the city. As the trail curves left, Rose Hill Cemetery is up a hill on the left. At this point, turn around to head back to your car.

NEARBY ATTRACTIONS

Take a few minutes while in downtown Rockmart to pay your respects to the citizens of the town who fought in American wars, including both World Wars, the Korean War, and the Vietnam War. The moving memorial before the city hall is only a few steps from the Rockmart trailhead.

SPRINGER MOUNTAIN LOOP TRAIL 25

IN BRIEF

This trail combines the start of the Appalachian Trail and the Benton MacKaye Trail to form a loop that begins (and ends) at the popular FS 42 parking lot.

DESCRIPTION

The Appalachian Trail (A.T.) is a 2,000-plus-mile hiking adventure from Maine to Georgia that many people start but few finish. Benton MacKaye conceived the idea of a trail along the eastern ridge of the Appalachian Mountains in 1921 after hiking Vermont's Long Trail. MacKaye, a Harvard-educated forester, left the Appalachian Trail Conference in the 1930s and formed the Wilderness Society with a group of fellow conservationists.

Directions ⟶

Take I-75 North to Exit 268, I-575. At the border between Cherokee and Pickens counties, I-575 becomes GA 515, also called the Georgia Mountain Parkway. Travel north 22.6 miles to GA 52, just north of Ellijay. Turn left (east) onto GA 52 at the end of the ramp. At 6.8 miles turn left onto Roy Road at Stanley's Chevron. At 4.3 miles Roy Road makes a hard left. At 6.6 miles there is a stop sign at Old Bucktown Road. Go straight. At 6.9 miles Roy Road makes another hard left at Parker Road. At 9.4 miles Roy Road dead-ends into Doublehead Gap Road, although the road is unmarked. Bear right and continue on Doublehead Gap Road. Pleasant Hill Baptist Church is 2.1 miles down on the left, and the signed entrance to Blue Ridge Wildlife Management Area of the Chattahoochee National Forest is on the right. Turn right on Forest Service Road (FS) 42 and travel 6.5 miles to the day-use parking area for Appalachian Trail Springer Mountain on the left. Walk to the brown-roofed building in the northwest corner of the parking lot.

KEY AT-A-GLANCE INFORMATION

LENGTH: 4.4 miles

CONFIGURATION: Loop

DIFFICULTY: Moderate, mostly because of the rocky uphill climb to Springer Mountain

SCENERY: Long-distance views into the Amicalola River watershed from Springer Mountain and into the Etowah River watershed from Ball Mountain

EXPOSURE: Mostly shaded

TRAFFIC: Heavy from the parking area to Springer Mountain; the Benton MacKaye portion of the trail is lightly used

TRAIL SURFACE: Compact dirt

HIKING TIME: 3 hours

ACCESS: Open year-round

MAPS: Fannin County Chamber of Commerce, phone (800) 899-6867; USGS Noontootla, Amicalola

FACILITIES: Primitive outhouse at Springer Mountain Shelter

SPECIAL COMMENTS: In April you may run into colorful Appalachian Trail through-hikers.

UTM Trailhead Coordinates

UTM Zone (NAD27) 16S

Easting   0757093

Northing   3836197

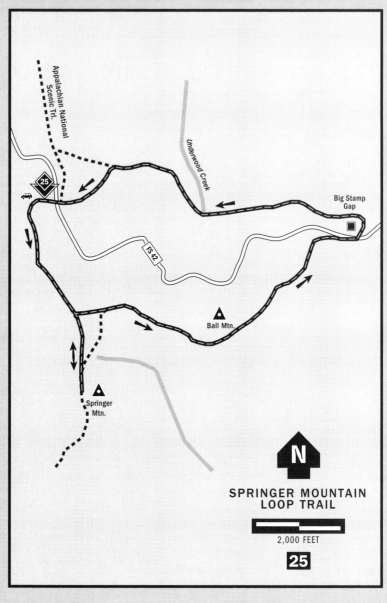

Appalachian National Scenic Trl.

Underwood Creek

25

FS 42

Big Stamp Gap

Ball Mtn.

Springer Mtn.

N

SPRINGER MOUNTAIN LOOP TRAIL

2,000 FEET

25

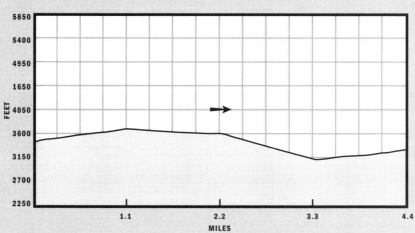

5850
5400
4950
1650
4050
3600
3150
2700
2250

FEET

1.1   2.2   3.3   4.4

MILES

When the Georgia portion of the hike was originally laid out, it extended to Mount Oglethorpe, near Jasper. There were many problems with the final 15 miles of the original hike, so the end of the trail was rerouted to Springer Mountain, which was in the Chattahoochee National Forest. Additionally, as a result of this rerouting, Amicalola Falls could serve as the access point for long-distance hikers.

Originally known as Penitentiary Mountain, the name "Springer" probably comes from one of two sources: John Springer, the first Presbyterian to be ordained minister in Georgia (in 1790), or William G. Springer, an early settler of Carroll County, Georgia. Whichever man was so honored, the name began to appear near the start of the 20th century. In 1959 the Georgia A.T. Club rerouted the end of the Appalachian Trail to Springer Mountain.

Twenty years later the Benton MacKaye Trail Association (BMTA) was formed to create a trail along the western ridge of the Appalachians, also beginning at Springer Mountain and running through Georgia and Tennessee. Through 2004 the BMTA had completed more than 90 of the 250 planned trail miles. Two more intersections with the A.T. are planned, both in the Great Smoky Mountains National Park.

From the brown trailhead kiosk in the FS 42 parking lot, walk to the left, crossing the lot, go down a set of wooden steps, and cross FS 42. As the pathway reenters the woods, the forest is predominately oak, tulip poplar, and American beech. Watch for holly and hemlock in this mountain forest. Almost immediately, the Appalachian Trail begins a moderate climb along a ridge to the peak of Springer Mountain. The familiar white rectangular blaze is used throughout to mark the Appalachian Trail. On the right is the first of a number of good views into the Amicalola/Coosa River watershed.

An eight-foot rock wall at 0.2 miles is adjacent to Springer Mountain Loop. Just past the wall is a tree that animals hollowed out and occasionally populate. Continuing on the A.T., you'll get additional long-distance views that are perhaps best in the winter and early spring. In this area, rock-lined culverts have been carefully crafted to move water away from the rocky, rooted trail. At the marked intersection with the Benton MacKaye Trail on the left, continue straight ahead toward Springer Mountain.

A second trail, also on the left, takes overnight hikers to the Springer Mountain Shelter. Continue straight ahead to the top of the mountain. The trail winds through a boulder-strewn area then comes out on solid rock with an unimpeded long-distance view to the southwest, making it an excellent place to watch the sunset. Two markers indicate the start of the Appalachian Trail: one features a 1930s-style hiker, courtesy of the Georgia A.T. Club, and another shows a map of the trail, courtesy of the U.S. Forest Service.

After spending a few minutes enjoying the view, return to the white diamond–blazed Benton MacKaye Trail, turn right, and begin an easy descent as the trail follows the curve of the mountain. In less than 0.1 mile, embedded in a rock on your right is a memorial plaque that tells hikers about the legacy of the trail's namesake. An easy-to-moderate ascent marks the start of Ball Mountain, which the Benton MacKaye skirts just beneath the peak. As the trail begins its descent to Big Stamp Gap, winter views through a deciduous forest off to the right at 2 miles into the hike foreshadow the scenic highlight of the trail at 2.4 miles. About 200 feet down a marked side trail is an excellent view of the northeast Georgia mountains.

Crossing FS 42 at 2.8 miles into the hike, the trail continues downhill, making a sweeping turn to the left and running parallel to but beneath the Forest Service road. Repeatedly, the trail runs through rhododendron thickets that are so full they actually form a canopy over the trail, protecting it from the hot summer sun. The first canopy, at 3.1 miles, indicates that a stream is paralleling the trail on the left side. The trail makes a wet-foot crossing of the stream at 3.3 miles. Over the next 0.3 miles, the path crosses streams twice, and there are a couple of low-light opportunities to photograph cascades near the trail. Turn left on the A.T. at the signed intersection at 4 miles and return to the parking lot on FS 42.

NEARBY ATTRACTIONS

Ellijay is home to the Georgia Apple Festival, which occurs on the second and third full weekends in October). You can buy anything made from an apple at the festival, or simply browse the shops on Winesap Way or Grannie Smith Street. For more information, call the Gilmer County Chamber of Commerce at (706) 635-7400, Monday through Friday.

TALKING ROCK NATURE TRAIL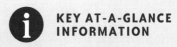

IN BRIEF

One of four developed trails in the Carters Lake area, this footpath takes hikers to a stunning overlook of Carters Lake reregulation pool and Georgia's Valley and Ridge section.

DESCRIPTION

Talking Rock Nature Trail begins as a short, moderate downhill hike through two brown posts placed to exclude vehicles. The trail moderates as it bears left, making a U-turn deep in a forested cove. On the left, after the turn, is an area that has been cleared and replanted with trees and shrubs designed to attract wildlife, including deer, squirrel, turkey, and songbirds. The trail is interpreted, with signs pointing out some of the improvements that have been made.

Past the feeding area, the trail bears right, following a small creek on the right down to a three-trail intersection. Straight ahead is a park bench, with a view of an area designed to attract wood ducks. Nearly extinct at the start of the

---

Directions ⟶

Take GA 515 North to GA 136. Turn left and immediately get in the right-turn lane. At 0.1 mile turn right on GA 136. Get in the left lane, drive 0.2 miles, and bear left. At 2.1 miles turn right on GA 136 at Bart's Bait and Tackle. Travel 10 miles, turning right at the visitor center sign. Bear left at 1.9 miles (the road to the right is for the visitor center). The guard shack is directly in front of you. Pay a $4 entrance fee, which allows you access to the North Bank Recreation Area, including this trail, the dam overlook, and a picnic area. Trail parking is 0.2 miles on the left. Look for an overhead Talking Rock Nature Trail sign 20 feet down the hill.

KEY AT-A-GLANCE INFORMATION

LENGTH: 2.4 miles

CONFIGURATION: Balloon

DIFFICULTY: Moderate

SCENERY: Excellent long-distance views into Georgia's Valley and Ridge section, and of the reregulation pool for Carters Lake. Continue into the North Bank Recreation Area for lakeside views of Carters Lake, the powerhouse channel, and the dam.

EXPOSURE: Mostly shaded, except toward the overlook, where the trail enters full sun

TRAFFIC: Moderate

TRAIL SURFACE: Compacted soil

HIKING TIME: 1.25 hours

ACCESS: Open year-round, dawn–dusk

MAPS: Carters Lake map available at the visitor center (right-hand turn before the trail); USGS Oakman

FACILITIES: None on trail; restrooms at visitor center

SPECIAL COMMENTS: This trail has plenty of wildlife, especially deer. You will need to wear hunter's orange during deer season (September–November).

UTM Trailhead Coordinates

UTM Zone (NAD27) 16S

Easting 0714106

Northing 3831965

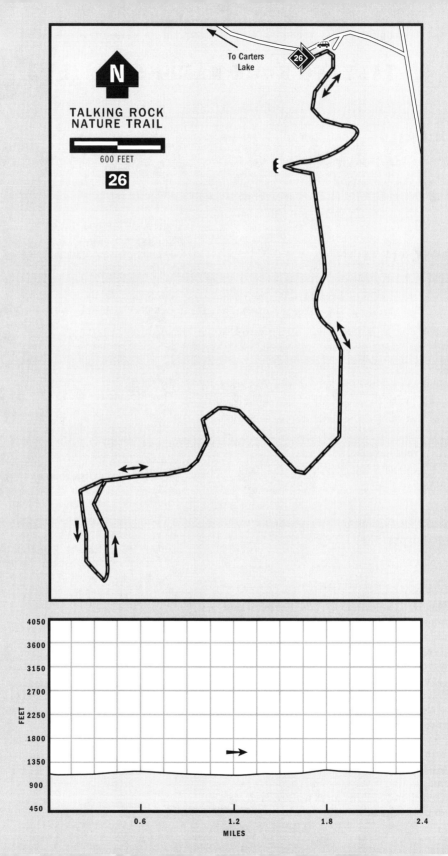

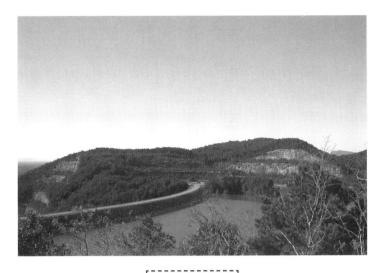

Carters Lake Dam

20th century, the wood duck was protected by treaty in 1918. It has had a long, slow recovery in both Georgia and the nation as a whole. Today the bird is no longer protected, but the species is closely watched in Georgia because much of its native habitat is being destroyed by development. Continue past the bench to a man-made rock dam that formed the small lake specifically designed to create wood duck habitat. Turn around and return to the three-way intersection.

At the intersection, turn right on a gravel road covered with mulch. On the right is the river that was dammed to form the lake; on the left is a moderate ascent to an unnamed knob. Note the large trees, some of which are oak, in the bottomland forest on the right. Two things important to creating wood duck habitat are mature oak (wood ducks feed on acorns) and forested wetlands (habitat).

Trees are typical Blue Ridge Mountain mix, with post and white oak; American beech; some hickory, pin oak, and red maple; occasional shortleaf and loblolly pine; and holly. As the fully shaded trail climbs through the forest, the valley on the right levels and widens. At 0.7 miles the gentle valley on the right ends and a steep-sided valley forms immediately on the left. This area is a known buck scrape, and hikers need to be careful here, especially during hunting season. Wear hunter's orange between September and November.

The wide path is easy over the next 0.2 miles, but as you enter an area the southern pine beetle has extensively destroyed, the path begins a moderate descent to an intersection with a trail that heads off to the left. Bear right and continue to a second intersection, which marks the start of the overlook loop. Pine beetle devastation is still apparent here, but the trail slowly regains trees as it comes around to the west side of the mountain.

The trees soon open up, letting you see the reregulation pool directly in front of and beneath you. From this overlook, the rolling hills of Georgia's Valley

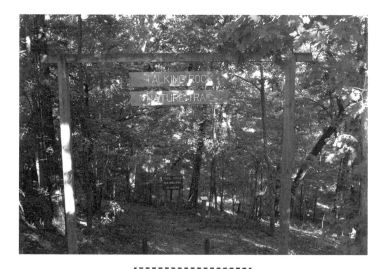

Talking Rock Trailhead

and Ridge section not only create a beautiful scene but also represent a major geologic division of the state. You are standing on the Blue Ridge Mountains, metamorphic rock formed during an uplift some 350 million years ago, looking out on a much older formation of sedimentary rock, indicating that the region was once covered by a great inland sea.

Carters Lake, which reached its full level for the first time in 1977, destroyed some of the finest whitewater runs in the nation. It was here that the outdoorsman and poet James Dickey had a real-life run-in with moonshiners that led him to write *Deliverance*. The reregulation dam was added to allow water to pass through the generators at peak hours and then be pumped back into the lake during off-peak hours, efficiently getting the maximum power out of every cubic foot of water.

From the overlook the path continues, curving to the left beside an open field and eventually returning to the start of the loop. Turn left and follow the path back to the starting point.

NEARBY ATTRACTIONS

Add the nearby Hidden Pond Songbird Trail to this hike as a good cool-down. This bird habitat is a nearby easy hike of 0.6 miles. To reach the trailhead, return to GA 136, then turn right and travel 1 mile to old US 411. Turn right and travel 0.4 miles to South Reregulation Dam Park. Follow the road around to the parking area; a large brown sign marks the trailhead.

THREE FORKS LOOP TRAIL 27

IN BRIEF

The Three Forks Loop combines portions of the Appalachian Trail and the Benton Mac-Kaye Trail between the day-use parking lot on FS 42 and Three Forks.

DESCRIPTION

This rugged, remote trail is a great place to get away from it all, quite literally. On the Thursday afternoon we hiked it, we did not meet a single person. Hunting is not permitted in the vicinity of the Appalachian Trail but is allowed along the Benton MacKaye, so wear hunter's orange between September and November (hunting season). A deeply creviced rock designed to block motorized vehicles marks the start of the trail. The white rectangular–blazed Appalachian Trail is straight ahead and

KEY AT-A-GLANCE INFORMATION

LENGTH: 6.6 miles

CONFIGURATION: Loop

DIFFICULTY: Moderate

SCENERY: Some long-distance winter views

EXPOSURE: Full shade

TRAFFIC: Light

TRAIL SURFACE: Packed clay

HIKING TIME: 3.5 hours

ACCESS: Open year-round

MAPS: USGS Noontootla; Fannin County Chamber of Commerce, phone (800) 899-MTNS (6867)

FACILITIES: None

SPECIAL COMMENTS: The original Appalachian Trail, which was rerouted in the 1970s, is now known as the Benton MacKaye Trail in this area.

Directions ⟶

From the end of I-575, take GA 515, also called the Georgia Mountain Parkway, 22.6 miles north to GA 52, just north of Ellijay. Turn left at the end of the ramp. At 6.8 miles turn left onto Roy Road, at Stanley's Chevron. At 4.3 miles Roy Road makes a hard left. At 6.6 miles there is a stop sign at Old Bucktown Road. Go straight. At 6.9 miles Roy Road makes another hard left at Parker Road. At 9.4 miles Roy Road dead-ends into Doublehead Gap Road, although the road is unmarked. Bear right and continue on Doublehead Gap Road. Pleasant Hill Baptist Church is 2.1 miles down on the left, and the signed entrance to Blue Ridge Wildlife Management Area of the Chattahoochee National Forest is on the right. Turn right on FS 42 and travel 6.5 miles to the Appalachian Trail Springer Mountain day-use parking area, on the left. Walk to the brown-roofed building at the northwest corner of the parking lot.

UTM Trailhead Coordinates

UTM Zone (NAD27) 16S

Easting 0757133

Northing 3836290

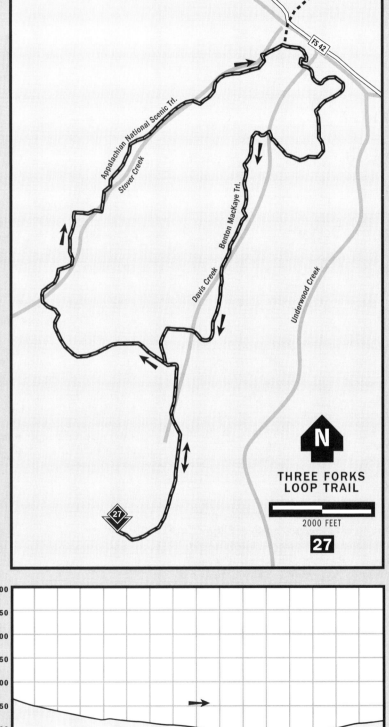

FS 42

Appalachian National Scenic Trl.

Stover Creek

Benton MacKaye Trl.

Davis Creek

Underwood Creek

N

**THREE FORKS
LOOP TRAIL**

2000 FEET

27

27

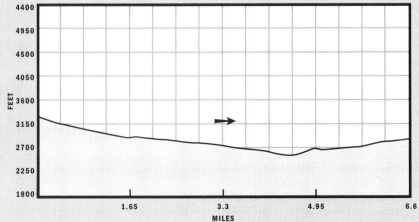

clearly marked. A level, grassy area off to the right after the rock may be confused with the trail, but it's short and goes nowhere.

Immediately entering a second-growth forest, where post, white, and pin oak predominate, with red maple and an occasional loblolly pine thrown in, you begin a long arc to the left around the top of a mountain. After you complete the arc, you'll see a large, moderately steep valley on your right. At just under 0.5 miles, you'll reach the first intersection with Benton MacKaye Trail. Go straight, following the Appalachian Trail through rhododendron thickets. These are known locally as laurel hells because the thickets are so thick that their common companion, mountain laurel, cannot grow. At times the rhododendron form an arch over the footpath. After a rain, Davis Creek, a tributary of Chester Creek, can be heard nearby.

Although the A.T. is poorly marked in this area, the path is well defined, continuing to curve around a mountain on your left. Davis Creek lies in front of you, a rooted, rocky, wet-foot crossing. About 25 feet after you cross Davis Creek, you'll reach a second creek, which runs after a heavy rainfall and may also have to be forded.

Now the path meanders into a laurel thicket (rhododendron hell) interspersed with tulip poplar and maturing evergreens. At 1 mile the A.T. again crosses Benton MacKaye Trail. This is the return point of the loop. Continue straight on the A.T. Until this point the footpath has been following near the top of a long ridge known as Rich Mountain. Now the A.T. comes off the ridge, falling, sometimes sharply, to the valley that holds Stover Creek.

As you descend the ridge, the sound of cascading water fills the air. In places, ferns indicate that the ground is regularly moist, and the trail becomes rooted and rocky. At 1.8 miles there is a good winter panorama of the valley that the A.T. follows. Continuing the descent, the trail reaches a set of ten rolled-log steps and a T-intersection. Turn left at the bottom of the steps. The path briefly follows an old logging road and then enters the forest, passing through a rhododendron thicket before steeply descending to Stover Creek. The trail to Stover Creek Shelter, a blue rectangular–blazed path, heads off to the left at 1.9 miles.

After crossing Stover Creek (a wet-thigh crossing) the trail climbs up the riverbank and back into the forest, quickly reaching a right turn on a road with a sign pointing to Three Forks. Over the next 1.5 miles, the footpath continues downhill much more gradually, with the occasional few steep steps. During this portion of the trek to Three Forks, the A.T. parallels Stover Creek, which is never more than 100 feet away.

In the Stover Creek valley, both the pathway and nearby areas tend to be moist, and at one point a tributary cascades onto the trail. Finally crossing Stover Creek on a bridge with handrails (the old bridge, a large log with one flat side, lies to the left), the A.T. begins to follow an old logging road. Just past the bridge, a side trail heads off to the left, and about 0.5 miles later Benton MacKaye Trail heads off to the right, marked with a wooden sign. Bear left and continue 0.1 mile on the A.T. to Three Forks, where Stover, Chester, and Long creeks form Noontootla Creek.

This area sees heavy use, and the lack of significant undergrowth near the crossing is a concern that will have to be addressed in the future. Turn around and return to the intersection with Benton MacKaye Trail, and turn left.

Named for the man who conceived the Appalachian Trail, at least in this area Benton MacKaye Trail follows the A.T.'s original path. MacKaye (rhymes with "eye") parted ways with members of the Appalachian Trail Club after a dispute and formed the Wilderness Society with other conservationists. Ultimately, the Benton MacKaye and Appalachian Trail will form a loop of nearly 500 miles through Georgia, North Carolina, and Tennessee.

As you turn onto the Benton MacKaye, it almost immediately enters a forest composed of pine saplings and rhododendron, with larger trees farther from the path. The trail begins an S-curve, climbing to an old road where it continues a moderate-to-difficult climb back to the top of Rich Mountain. On your left, a deep, steep-sided valley offers good winter views. The road circles the mountain as it climbs, finally leveling off as it approaches the top of Rich Mountain, where the road is blocked and the path bears right, into the forest.

Unlike the A.T. some 600 feet below, the Benton MacKaye crosses no rivers and shows little sign of moisture. Along the ridgetop the lightly used trail will narrow where grass encroaches. Luckily, the Benton MacKaye is well blazed, and you rarely take more than a few steps before seeing another blue-rectangle blaze indicating A.T. access or a white-diamond blaze of its own path.

Curving gracefully to the right but still climbing, the trail circles near the top of an unnamed knob then curves back to the left to continue its final ascent to Rich Mountain. At 4.6 miles you reach the mile-long ridge that is the top of Rich Mountain. Along the ridgetop the ascent continues at an easy grade, with only the occasional short level or downhill stretches. Finally, at 5.4 miles you reach the pinnacle of Rich Mountain. Over the next 0.3 miles, the Benton MacKaye makes an easy descent to the intersection with the A.T. Turn left on the A.T. and return to the day-use parking lot on FS 42.

NEARBY ATTRACTIONS

On your way to the trail, stop by Colonel Poole's to fill up on classic Georgia barbecue and see the Pig Hill of Fame. Open Friday through Sunday, 11 a.m. to 8 p.m., Colonel Poole's is adjacent to the Georgia Mountain Parkway in Ellijay. Turn right on Maddox Street, then make an immediate left.

VICKERY CREEK TRAIL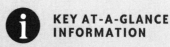

IN BRIEF

This loop trail explores a low knoll north of the Chattahoochee River east of the oxbow in Vickery Creek. The fast-moving creek supplied power to Roswell Mill, which you can also explore on this hike.

DESCRIPTION

Unlike most of the Chattahoochee River National Recreation Area hikes, the Vickery Creek hike does not explore the floodplain of the Chattahoochee River and does not approach the Chattahoochee itself. Rather, the hike covers a small knoll north of the river, along Vickery Creek, twice dipping to the broad, full river that once powered Roswell Cotton Mill and many other mills in the area.

This hike begins at the Oxbo Trail parking lot instead of the Vickery Creek Unit parking area because the small National Recreation Area lot is frequently full on weekends, and the single-lane entrance is dangerous. Follow Vickery Creek, which is also known as Big Creek, 0.3 miles until it curves left and rises slightly. At the top of the rise, turn right and climb the stairs to the bridge over the creek. On the left a dam-created waterfall is a pleasing sight at the start of the hike. On the far side of the bridge, the path bears left, climbing stairs as it curves back around to the right.

KEY AT-A-GLANCE INFORMATION

LENGTH: 6.5 miles

CONFIGURATION: Loop

DIFFICULTY: Moderate

SCENERY: Views of creek, antebellum dam, covered bridge, Roswell Mill

EXPOSURE: Partially shaded

TRAFFIC: Moderate

TRAIL SURFACE: Compacted dirt, some gravel

HIKING TIME: 3 hours

ACCESS: Open year-round, dawn–dusk

MAPS: On map stands throughout the hike, except for the portion near Roswell Mill; Chattahoochee River National Recreation Area (CRNRA) Headquarters at Island Ford; USGS Roswell

FACILITIES: None

SPECIAL COMMENTS: This diverse hardwood forest is more typical of the Georgia mountains farther north.

Directions

Take GA 400 North from Atlanta to Exit 6, Northridge Road. Travel 0.4 miles to GA 9/ Roswell Road and turn right at the light. Follow Roswell Road 4.9 miles to Oxbo Road. Turn right and travel 0.1 mile to the gravel parking lot on your right.

UTM Trailhead Coordinates

UTM Zone (NAD27) 16S

Easting   0744655

Northing   3765941

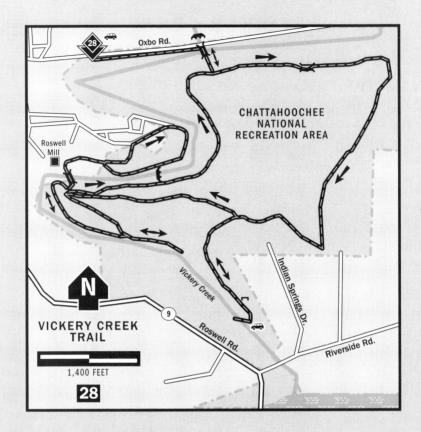

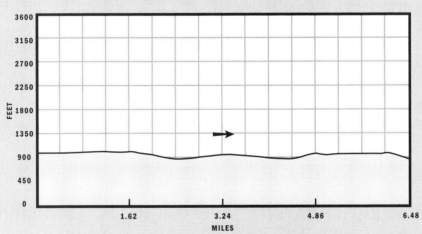

The familiar CRNRA entrance kiosk is on the left, with a "you are here" map on a separate pedestal.

Initially the trail continues its climb through a mature second-growth hardwood forest composed of post and white oak, and less frequently pin and red oak, normally dotted with loblolly and/or shortleaf pine. American beech, hickory, and sassafras are common in some areas. Red fox, wild turkey, beaver, otter, and tortoise are among the wildlife that can be spotted on this trail.

Coming to a T-intersection near the top of the unnamed knoll, turn left. The trail quickly begins an easy-to-moderate descent to a wet-foot crossing of a tributary of Vickery Creek. After a brief climb, the trail rolls through an area of pine beetle destruction to a second easy-to-moderate descent to the Grimes Bridge Road entrance kiosk at 0.8 miles into the hike. Turn right and begin climbing, once again through an area destroyed by the pine beetle.

The first of two major crossover trails heads off to the right at 1 mile; this is actually an old road that leads to Roswell Mill Dam (notice the road continues on the left, but this is not a path). As you continue on the main trail, notice that it, too, has become a road, covered with gravel in places. You can see houses off to the left; the second crossover trail heads off to the right at 1.1 miles. The footpath descends to a side trail to the left, and you soon reach an intrusive chain-link fence where the main trunk makes an abrupt right-hand turn into a climb at 1.4 miles. The path then heads past another side trail to the housing development and the three-way intersection with the trail from the CRNRA parking area. Turn left and follow the trail for an easy descent, with Vickery Creek gorge on the right. A side trail on the right went down to the cliffs, but this trail has been closed for many years.

Becoming a moderate descent, the footpath makes an unusual change at 1.8 miles. The rocky path becomes rock-free and graded for the next 0.1 mile, when an old road goes straight as the path bears right at a bench. Shortly past the bench the trail switches back and becomes steeper, finally dropping down a set of wooden steps at the entry to the river gorge. Down to the left is the CRNRA kiosk, to the right a brief path that quickly closes. We recommend you pay the $3 usage fee because most of the money stays locally and helps improve the federal parks in the Atlanta area. Turn around and retrace your steps to the main trunk and turn left.

With the river valley occasionally visible on the left, the footpath continues to rise to a crossover trail at 2.6 miles, quickly followed by a three-way intersection 0.1 mile later. Turn left and begin an easy descent into the Vickery Creek gorge. As the footpath approaches a left turn at 3 miles it becomes steeper, but never more than moderate. When the trail reaches the river, turn left and follow Vickery Creek past a sewer pipe until a wire blocks access to the cliffs, at 3.4 miles. Turn around and follow the river to the bend, stepping up and over another sewer pipe. As the trail makes a 90-degree right turn, Georgia's newest covered bridge comes into view. The path leads you under the bridge, but don't try to

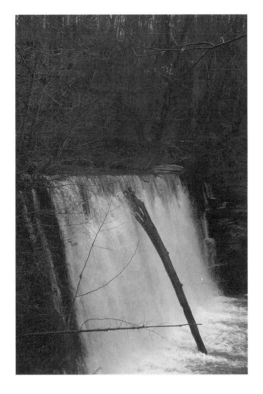

Sweetwater Creek Falls at the Brevard Fault Line

climb uphill near the bridge—there's a much easier way to get there.

Return to the three-way intersection and turn left, climbing back to the second intersection. Bear right (don't take the hard right, the trail you came in on), and watch on the left for the trail a few steps up the path. When we hiked this trail, it was only slightly discernible, but that was shortly after construction was complete. The trail drops steeply to the covered bridge, which spans Vickery Creek. On the far side, the trail climbs a gravel road, passing one of many buildings collectively known as Roswell Mill.

As the road reaches a level section, bear right and follow the path down to the mill's powerhouse and dam. Just before you reach the powerhouse, turn right and descend to the riverbank; follow this to a wooden viewing deck just before the dam.

Return to the trail and turn right, following the footpath to a gravel road that sharply rises to King's Mill Court, a paved residential street. Turn left on Sloan Street. As Founder's Cemetery appears on the right, the entrance to an interpreted trail leading to Roswell Mill is on the left, just after a small streetside parking lot. Descending the stairs, you'll find signs telling the story of Roswell Mill. As you return to the riverbank, turn right and retrace your steps to the covered bridge, climbing to the Vickery Creek Trail complex after crossing the bridge. Turn left and follow the wide path as it climbs to a road to the left at 5.5 miles. This road drops steadily to the milldam. This is a pleasant area for a break, with the roaring water of Vickery Creek tumbling over the massive dam.

Turn around and climb back to the top of the road and turn right. The trail becomes a footpath through thickets of mountain laurel and rhododendron. A three-way intersection is marked by a split-rail fence on the left to prevent hikers from trying to climb down the steep, fragile embankment to the mill dam. Continue straight, and the trail once again becomes a footpath through a sometimes dense forest. A stream with a couple of small waterfalls requires a wet-foot crossing at 5.9 miles as the footpath gently sweeps to the left. As Vickery Creek Trail curves back around to the right, it passes a crossover trail off to the right at 6 miles. From this point the trail drops quickly to the start of the loop, where you turn left and return to your car.

NEARBY ATTRACTIONS

Archibald Smith was an influential resident of Roswell. His 1840s plantation home is adjacent to the impressive Roswell City Hall and is open Monday through Friday (with tours at 11:30 a.m., 12:30 p.m., 1:30 p.m., and 2:30 p.m.) and Saturday (with tours at 10:30 a.m., 11:30 a.m., 12:30 p.m., and 1:30 p.m.). According to the city of Roswell, which owns the site, the home features original furnishings and 12 outbuildings. Turn left out of the parking lot, travel 0.1 mile to Roswell Road, turn right, and proceed 2 blocks to Hill Street. Make the first left into the city hall parking lot, and continue to the other side of the building. Watch for the signed entrance on the left.

29 WILD HORSE CREEK TRAIL

 KEY AT-A-GLANCE INFORMATION

LENGTH: 4 miles

CONFIGURATION: Out-and-back

DIFFICULTY: Easy

SCENERY: Long-distance views of the park-like setting, view of Noses Creek from trestle on Silver Comet Trail

EXPOSURE: Full sun

TRAFFIC: Moderate

TRAIL SURFACE: Concrete

HIKING TIME: 1.75 hours

ACCESS: Open year-round, dawn–dusk, except after a heavy rain

MAPS: USGS Lost Mountain, Austell

FACILITIES: Restrooms in Wild Horse Creek Park, solar-powered emergency phones on trail

SPECIAL COMMENTS: Watch for the largest red maple tree (authenticated by Georgia's Championship Trees Program) in the state near the Wild Horse Creek Park trailhead. When we measured it in 2007, the tree was 18 feet around.

UTM Trailhead Coordinates

UTM Zone (NAD27) 16S

Easting 0716257

Northing 3750648

IN BRIEF

This hike follows the level floodplain of Wild Horse Creek and Noses Creek to the Noses Creek Trestle, climbing at the finish to Silver Comet Trail.

DESCRIPTION

Wild Horse Creek Trail was the first planned side trail to Silver Comet Trail and is part of an exciting overall plan by the Cobb County Department of Transportation to provide a countywide system of greenways and parks. The trail, which is owned by the City of Powder Springs, is designed to connect Wild Horse Creek Park to Silver Comet Trail and the Cobb County greenway system.

Beginning on the east side of the trail's parking area, near a kiosk and a map stand provided by Powder Springs, the trail curves right to a three-way stop, crosses Macedonia Road, and then passes two houses on Lancer Drive. After the second house, the trail turns left and passes under a hanging garden, then turns right as it enters the floodplain of Wild Horse Creek.

Tributaries to Wild Horse Creek flow through culverts spanned by concrete bridges and iron-rail fences. The first of these is at 0.4 miles into the hike. At 0.6 miles a pullout with benches and a planting of river birch mark the

Directions

Take I-75 North to Exit 269 (GA 5/Ernest Barrett Parkway). At the end of the ramp, turn left and travel 10.6 miles to Macedonia Road. Turn right and drive 1.7 miles to the Wild Horse Creek Park Trail Parking area, just after a three-way stop. The trailhead is on the right after you enter the park.

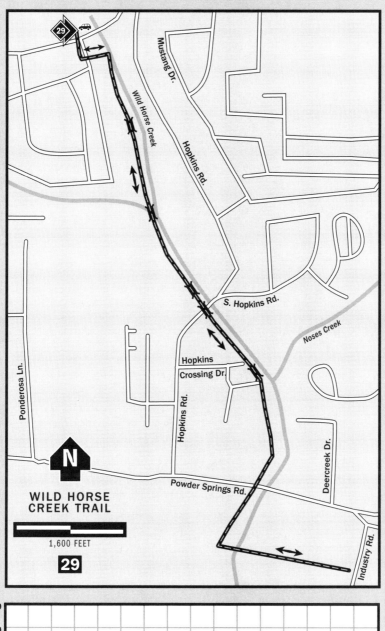

WILD HORSE
CREEK TRAIL

1,600 FEET

29

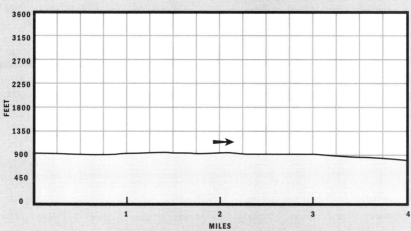

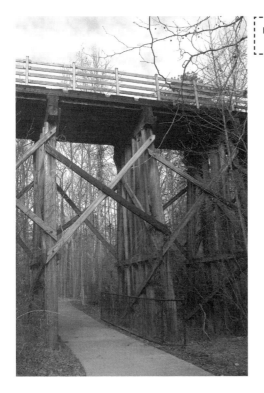

second tributary that joins Wild Horse Creek. Woody shrubs broken by occasional loblolly pines make up the majority of the forest in this area. The trail crosses another bridge on the approach to Hopkins Road, a traffic-light intersection.

After Hopkins Road, the trail begins to rise almost imperceptibly above the adjoining forested wetlands adjacent to the path. Undergrowth off the path increases noticeably, and a two-story wooden observation tower on the right allows hikers an interesting view from above. The wetlands were teeming with wildlife in the cool winter morning. We spotted Canada geese, squirrels, and a raccoon within 15 minutes here. Turning right and leaving the observation tower, the path quickly comes to the confluence of Wild Horse and Noses creeks. According to Georgia historian John Goff, Noses Creek derives its name from a Cherokee chief who lived on the creek. Powder Springs is a shortening of its original name, Gunpowder Springs, one of a number of naturally occurring springs in the area. The spring contained potassium nitrate, an essential ingredient in gunpowder.

Wild Horse Creek Trail passes under the Noses Creek overpass on Powder Springs Road to bypass this busy street. As you emerge from the overpass, there is an excellent long-distance view of the creek and its adjacent riparian zones. At 1.7 miles the massive Noses Creek Trestle looms across the river, and Wild Horse Creek Trail passes under the creosote wood bridge. After the trestle the trail makes a quick curve right, climbing up a good thigh-burning hill, then makes another hard right where it dead-ends into Silver Comet Trail. Turn right and walk to the trestle, which is only a few steps down the path. As you cross the trestle, take a few minutes to study both the creek and the diverse forest in its floodplain from above. White, post, and red oak; American beech; and various pines form the majority of the forest.

Take a few minutes and walk along the old rail bed that is now known as Silver Comet Trail. Scheduled to be more than 50 miles long, crossing the counties west of Atlanta, Silver Comet Trail stretches 12.8 miles in Cobb County. On

Pond overlook on Wild Horse Creek Trail

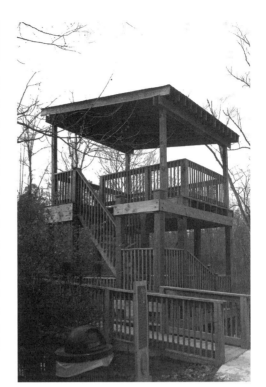

the western end it will join Chief Ladiga Trail in Alabama, creating a continuous trail from Smyrna, Georgia, to Anniston, Alabama. Two other hikes feature portions of this trail, Silver Comet Trail: Mavell Road to Floyd Road and Silver Comet Trail: Rockmart. After passing under some high-tension power lines, turn around at Industry Road, near a microwave tower and natural gas facility. Follow the Silver Comet back over the Noses Creek Trestle and continue on to Carter Road. Turn around, return to the Wild Horse Trail entrance, and retrace your steps to the trailhead.

NEARBY ATTRACTIONS

Follow Macedonia Road west 0.1 mile and turn right to enter the main area of Wild Horse Creek Park. The park features picnic areas, a playground, and a BMX bike track.

30 WILDCAT CREEK TRAIL

 KEY AT-A-GLANCE INFORMATION

LENGTH: 3 miles
CONFIGURATION: Out-and-back
DIFFICULTY: Easy–moderate
SCENERY: Views of Wildcat Creek
EXPOSURE: Mostly shaded
TRAFFIC: Light
TRAIL SURFACE: Packed dirt, gravel roads
HIKING TIME: 1.5 hours
ACCESS: Open year-round
MAPS: USGS Amicalola, Nelson
FACILITIES: None
SPECIAL COMMENTS: Although the trail is in a remote area of North Georgia, don't worry about wildcats; the name probably refers to the miners who sought alluvial gold.

UTM Trailhead Coordinates

UTM Zone (NAD27) 16S

Easting   0749568

Northing 3820455

IN BRIEF

This trail climbs into the Amicalola Creek watershed along Wildcat Creek. Because of the trail's remote nature, it is possible to see a wide range of wildlife.

DESCRIPTION

Although this portion of the Dawson Forest Wildlife Management Area is technically under the control of the Georgia Department of Natural Resources (DNR), it is the Mountain Stewards who have developed the multiple-trail complex in this area. Wildcat Tract spans the forest from Monument Road to Steve Tate Road, and the Mountain Stewards have developed Tobacco Pouch Trail, Fall Creek Trail, Rocky Ford Trail, Windy Ridge Trail, Turner Trail, and Wildcat Trail, a total of 12 miles of trails. For this hike we chose Wildcat Trail.

At the end of the Wildcat Campground, a brown hiker sign in front of the fast-flowing Amicalola River marks the trailhead. Follow the river 20 steps to the right to reach the first green blaze, which marks Wildcat Trail. Walk 0.1 mile to reach a wooden bridge built by the Mountain Stewards and the DNR. Take the bridge across the river and hike over some soggy level ground to reach Wildcat Creek.

Directions

Take I-575 North. At Ball Ground the road becomes SR 515, the Georgia Mountain Parkway. Turn right on SR 53. Continue 8.6 miles to Steve Tate Highway. Turn left and travel 7.2 miles on Steve Tate Highway to Wildcat Campground Road. Note: Steve Tate Highway becomes Steve Tate Road. Turn left and travel 0.8 miles to the campground. Follow the road to the far end of the campground and park on either side.

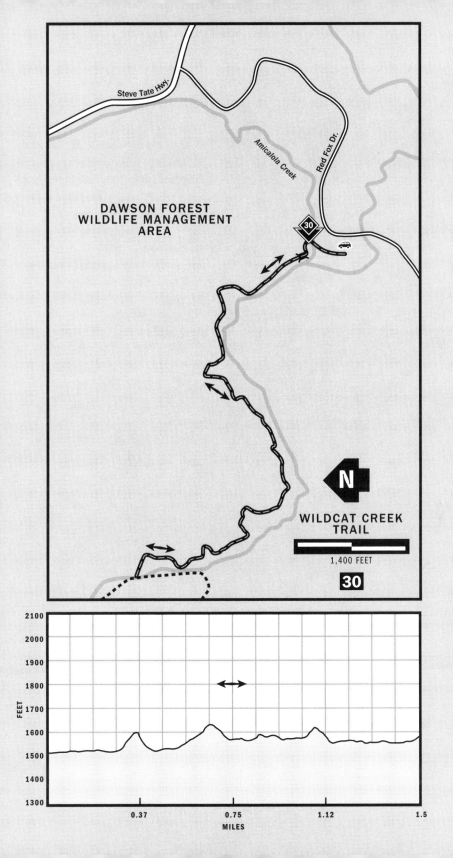

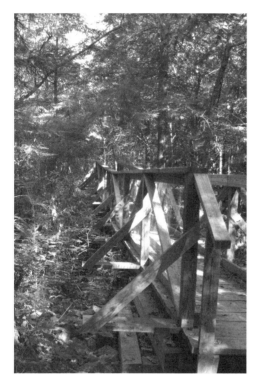

Bridge over Amicalola Creek

Follow it upstream into the watershed of the Amicalola River. Rhododendron is prevalent, as are shortleaf and longleaf pine, and hemlock. A variety of oak and dogwood abound near the trail that hugs a riverbank, which drops sharply to the creek. Occasionally, side trails allow access for fishing.

About 0.3 miles into the hike, the trail bears away from the river and begins climbing a small hill rising some 80 feet above the water. Climbing to the top is relatively easy, but the path narrows at the top, so returning to the river is a scramble down a steep, slippery, tree-rooted path with rock outcrops. As you return to the creek, rhododendron and laurel battle for sunlight, and both the river and trail make a 90-degree left-hand turn about 0.5 miles into the hike.

Joining an old road at 0.6 miles, the trail bears right (away from the river) and climbs into a mostly pine forest. Near the top of this hill, look left to see the river, well below you. As we climbed the third mountain, we heard the call of a hawk—not above us but to our left. He flew away with dinner—a grey squirrel—in his grasp. A short time later, we spotted the squirrel carcass a few feet off the trail. Leaving this hill the trail returned to the creek at 1.4 miles, now more heavily covered with rhododendron and requiring we carefully step over slippery rocks. Finally, 0.1 mile later, the trail ends at Wildcat Creek.

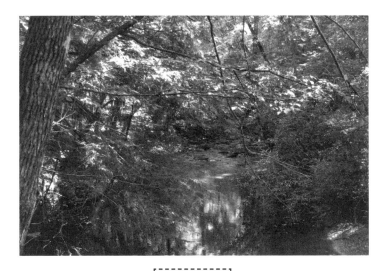

Wildcat Creek

NEARBY ATTRACTIONS

Any one of the trails in the Dawson Forest would be an excellent choice to add to this hike. For more information on these hikes, visit the Mountain Stewards Web site at **www.mountainstewards.org.**

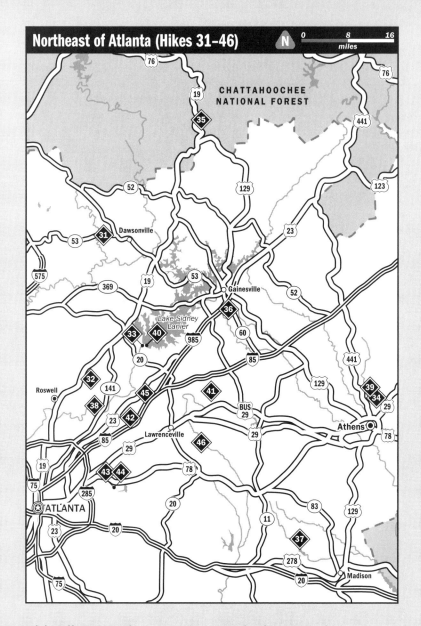

CHATTAHOOCHEE
NATIONAL FOREST

Dawsonville

Gainesville

Lake Sidney Lanier

Roswell

Lawrenceville

Athens

ATLANTA

Madison

NORTHEAST OF ATLANTA

31 AMICALOLA FALLS LOOP TRAIL

KEY AT-A-GLANCE INFORMATION

LENGTH: 2.8 miles

CONFIGURATION: Loop

DIFFICULTY: Difficult

SCENERY: Waterfalls, mountains

EXPOSURE: Full sun at the falls, visitor center, and along the upper third of the East Ridge; mostly shaded elsewhere

TRAFFIC: Heavy

TRAIL SURFACE: Compacted soil and gravel road. The trail from the West Ridge Parking Lot to the falls is made of rubber tires.

HIKING TIME: 2 hours

ACCESS: Closed Mondays, except legal holidays

MAPS: Available at visitor center; USGS Nimblewill, Amicalola

FACILITIES: Restrooms; wheelchair-accessible trails, including access to the falls; picnic tables; visitor center. Amicalola Falls is also the only access point to the southern terminus of the A.T. that allows long-term parking for thru-hikers. Amicalola Lodge is a renowned hotel. Hike Inn offers hikers who prefer a soft bed and good food

SPECIAL COMMENTS: The best views are after a winter rain, when there is no tree cover and the river flow is high

UTM Trailhead Coordinates

UTM Zone (NAD27) 16S

Easting 0756316

Northing 3812840

IN BRIEF

This trail explores the watershed of the Amicalola River in the area of Amicalola Falls.

DESCRIPTION

Tumbling 729 feet in a series of freefalls and large cascades, Amicalola Falls is clearly the focus of this trail. The first written account of these falls at the southern end of the Blue Ridge Mountains appeared in 1832 when surveyor William Williamson wrote, "I discovered a Water Fall perhaps the greatest in the World." Williamson was surveying lots for the Sixth Georgia Land Lottery, which precipitated the Cherokee Trail of Tears.

When the Appalachian Trail (A.T.) was rerouted to end at Springer Mountain in 1959, Amicalola Falls became known to most hikers as the southern terminus access for thru-hikers. A portion of the loop trail is actually part of the access trail, an 8-mile point-to-point path from Amicalola Falls to the A.T. trailhead on Springer Mountain.

Descending a set of stone steps from the parking lot, on the left you'll see interpretive

----

Directions

Take GA 400 North to GA 53 (at the first traffic light after the outlet mall). Turn left and travel 6.8 miles to a stop sign. Turn left and continue on GA 53 around Dawson County Courthouse and through downtown Dawsonville. Drive 2.7 miles and go right on GA 183, the Elliot Family Parkway. Travel 10.5 miles to GA 52, following the traffic triangle to the right. Travel 1.6 miles to the entrance to Amicalola Falls State Park and pay the $3 entrance fee. Just over 0.2 miles into the park, turn left onto Amicalola Lodge Road and travel 1.1 miles to the parking area on the right. If the lot is full, there is overflow parking down the road on the right.

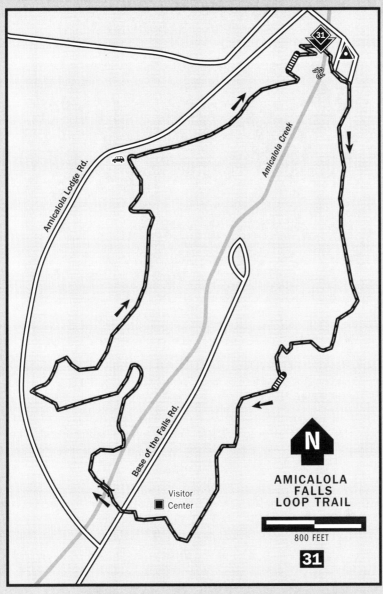

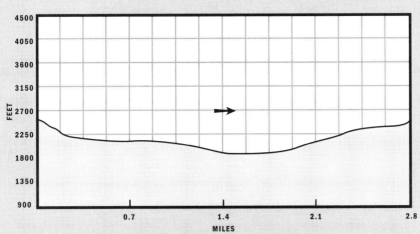

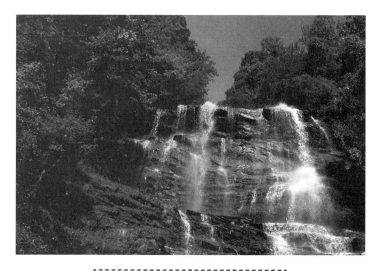

The "Tumbling Waters" of Amicalola Falls

signs discussing Hurricane Opal, which swept through the north Georgia Mountains on October 4, 1995. As you continue, the concrete path turns to wood, then juts out over the falls as the trees open up to reward you with a stunning view of the foothills of the southern Blue Ridge Mountains and the Amicalola River watershed. The stable flow of the Amicalola River, combined with its high oxygen content, makes the river an excellent fishing stream and provides habitat for a wide range of animals and waterfowl downstream.

Continue across the bridge, climbing a set of railed concrete steps to the paved east overflow parking area. Turn right, descending to the gated entrance to the East Ridge Trail. On your right are concrete block bathrooms and vending machines. The upper portion of East Ridge Trail follows the original gravel road to the top of Amicalola Falls. The upper portion of the road is sunny, rocky, and heavily rutted in areas, but the view to the right across the Georgia piedmont is simply stunning.

As the gravel road reenters the forest at 0.4 miles, the trail moderates. Now walking in partial shade through a mature second-growth hardwood forest, you'll find that the incline lessens and the road is less rutted. A double-blaze indicates a turn ahead, which comes at 0.5 miles at a red visitor-center sign. The trail descends wooden steps into the full shade of a deciduous forest composed of varieties of oak, native dogwood, and mountain laurel. Entering a cove at 0.7 miles, the trail traverses a gulley on a wooden boardwalk. Here the maturing hardwoods are beginning to take on the appearance of an old-growth forest.

Amicalola Falls Loop descends fieldstone steps at 1.1 miles into the opening for the visitor center. On the left is a stone in the shape of the State of Georgia, inscribed with the words "Maine to Georgia," the slogan for the A.T. Just past the stone is a stone bridge and an arch. You can walk around the building to the left (the restrooms are here), or enter the visitor center, which has displays on the natural history of the area, and an excellent bookstore. There are frequent ranger-led interpretive lessons at the center as well.

Cross the paved road to a small parking lot. At the far end of the lot is a wooden bridge over Amicalola Creek. On the far side of the bridge, the trail turns right and begins a steady, moderate climb; some 150 feet above the creek, there are occasional streamside views. Creek Trail ends at West Ridge Loop (1.5 miles). Turn left at the signed three-way intersection. Gradually climbing a gravel road for 0.2 miles, the trail bears right, returning to a forest of pine mixed with young oak. As the green-blazed trail rises, it comes to a confusing three-way intersection at 1.7 miles. All the trails sport the green blaze. Turn right here and continue your easy climb through a thicket of mountain laurel, which sometimes forms a canopy over the path.

Take the yellow-blazed Spring Trail that heads off to the left at 2 miles and begin a steady, moderate climb to the West Ridge parking area. The trail switch-backs a couple of times to ease the climb, and at 2.2 miles climbs a set of stairs, turns right, and then makes a left, following a grade to the embankment of the modern road. For a few steps, the pathway climbs on the embankment, then switches back and returns to compacted soil. Spring Trail ascends a set of stairs to the West Ridge parking lot. In the lot, turn right and continue to West Ridge Falls Access Trail. This easy, level trail is only 0.2 miles long and allows wheelchair access to the Lower Falls. At the end of this trail, a wooden bridge crosses in front of the falls, allowing visitors an unrivaled view of Amicalola Creek tumbling down the mountain. Return 0.1 mile to the metal grate stairs on your left.

The final ascent of the face of the falls requires hikers climb more than 300 steps, but there are wide areas with benches there for tired hikers. At the top of the stairs, turn right to return to the first long-distance view over the falls, or turn left to return to your car.

NEARBY ATTRACTIONS

For seasonal fun in the autumn, try Burt's Pumpkin Farm, across the street from the entrance to Amicalola Falls. Kids will love choosing their Halloween pumpkin, and Mom and Dad will have a good time creating memories. Phone (706) 265-3701.

32 BIG CREEK TRAIL

KEY AT-A-GLANCE INFORMATION

LENGTH: 12.5 miles

CONFIGURATION: Out-and-back with a balloon at the end

DIFFICULTY: Easy

SCENERY: Creekside views, forested wetlands

EXPOSURE: Partly shaded

TRAFFIC: Heavy

TRAIL SURFACE: Concrete pavement, except on the balloon at the end

HIKING TIME: 5 hours

ACCESS: Open year-round, dawn–dusk

MAPS: Brochure at trailhead (sometimes); USGS Roswell

FACILITIES: Restrooms near the end of the trail. Facilities at the start of the trail burned down but are being rebuilt.

SPECIAL COMMENTS: Atlanta's most cosmopolitan trail—it is possible to hear a wide variety of languages as you hike this trail with people from around the world.

UTM Trailhead Coordinates

UTM Zone (NAD27) 16S

Easting 0753425

Northing 3773079

IN BRIEF

This multiuse trail explores the floodplain of Big Creek (Vickery Creek) from Webb Bridge Road to Mansell Road.

DESCRIPTION

Rob Warrilow got the idea for Big Creek Trail when he visited his son at college in Colorado, where a similar trail existed. Warrilow, an engineer for the city of Alpharetta, knew that an easement in the hundred-year floodplain of Big Creek would be a great place to build the same kind of trail. He walked the Colorado trail with his video camera and returned to show the film to the city council as he discussed plans for the floodplain. With their support, Warrilow secured funding, and work on the trail began. The north and south ends were completed first. In 2001 the city completed the connection, creating a 6.2-mile-long park. Plans to extend the trail from Forsyth County to Cobb County (a total of 26 miles) were announced in 2005, and some work has begun.

From Greenways Parking, turn left on the sidewalk, crossing a side street that leads to parking for the YMCA youth camp. On the far side of the street, the path slowly drops into the surprisingly large Big Creek floodplain. On the left, the modern YMCA building

Directions ⟶

Take GA 400 North to Exit 10, Old Milton Highway. Turn right at end of the ramp and move to the left lane. At 0.6 miles turn left on Northpoint Parkway, travel 0.4 miles, and make a right on Preston Ridge Road. On-road parking is 0.1 mile down on the right. There is additional parking in Northpoint Mall and on Haynes Bridge Road next to the mall.

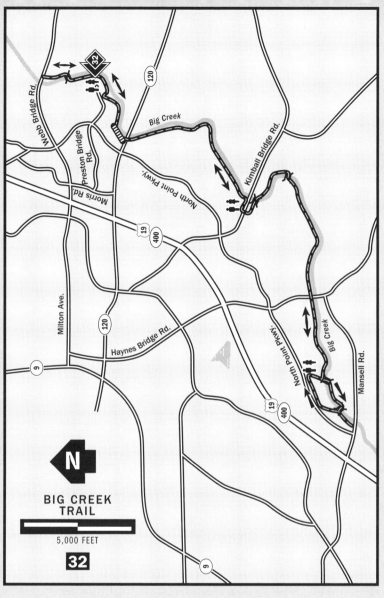

**BIG CREEK
TRAIL**

5,000 FEET

32

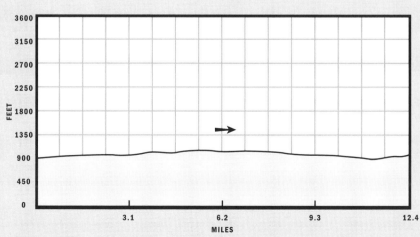

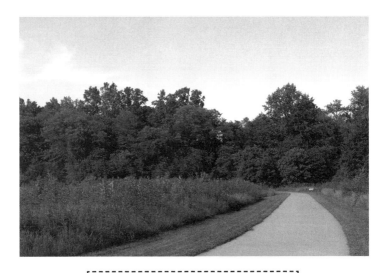

Big Creek Trail has little change in elevation.

rises well above the path. Post oak, river birch, and sycamore fill in the area between the trail and the river on the right side of the path. Just under 0.5 miles into the hike, Big Creek comes into view for the first time. Wide and fast flowing, its water is frequently muddy because of erosion, which is causing some concern. Urban runoff has also become a problem for the river, which provides some of the drinking water for communities along it.

A few steps farther on, the pathway curves right, crosses its first bridge—also concrete with metal railings—and curves left. On the right is a dirt path that goes to a hike-and-bike trail that adds 1 mile to the trip. The trail ends, at least for the time being, at Webb Bridge Road (at 0.8 miles). Turn around and retrace the route to the entrance, but as you cross the asphalt road, make a left. The YMCA youth camp area is on the left—the trail runs beside it as it drops gently before curving right. Be careful here because you can't see around the corner, and occasionally cyclists exceed the posted 10 mph speed limit. The trail runs next to apartments from here to Old Milton Highway. At 1.8 miles there is a small falls along the river to your left. Just over 2 miles into the hike, Big Creek Greenway makes an S-curve as a concrete stairway rises to Old Milton on the right. Following the stairway, the trail curves left under the Old Milton overpass, affording some good views of the creek at a metal railing.

A second bridge carries you across a tributary at 2.5 miles, where you'll see commercial buildings on the right and homes on the left. From this point on, you can sometimes see homes from the trail. As the trail curves around to the right at 3 miles, there is a forested wetlands on the right. A bridge over a tributary at 3.4 miles is followed by a concrete path heading off to the right, leading 0.5 miles to more commercial buildings. We spotted a pair of owls here, who joined us for part of the southbound walk. As the path makes a hard right, it begins rising to

Kimball Bridge Road, which it crosses at a controlled intersection. Next, the trail turns left, descends to Big Creek's floodplain, passes a wetlands marked "environmentally sensitive area," then crisscrosses the river. With Big Creek again on your left, the path makes a sweeping curve to the right and changes from a north–south trail to an east–west one. At 5.1 miles a trail on the right leads to a housing development, and then Big Creek Greenway arrives at the Haynes Bridge Road overpass 0.4 miles later. On the right is a trail to a parking area.

Splitting at 5.8 miles, the two paths come together 0.1 mile later. You'll soon reach a side path on the left that crosses Big Creek on a bridge and ends in a commercial area. At a four-way intersection at 6.3 miles, take the trail on the right 0.2 miles to the restrooms. Just before the restrooms, a wood chip–covered path heads off to the left, entering a mostly pine forest at the start of an extensive forested wetlands area. The trail turns left after a bridge at 6.7 miles, running beside Northpoint Mall for a short distance. As the trail curves back around to the right, there is a frequently muddy area followed by a side trail to another shopping area. At 7 miles the pathway turns into a boardwalk leading to a bridge over a creek. A trail heads off to the right as you step off the bridge; continue straight. The footpath climbs concrete steps up to the greenway. At this intersection you can go straight or left—they both return you to the previous four-way. We prefer the path on the left, which combines paved path, railed boardwalk, and an excellent scenic view into the forested wetlands to create a pleasant walk back to the four-way intersection. At the intersection take a few moments to view Big Creek from the bridge on your right. Return to the main trail, turn right, and retrace your steps to the car.

NEARBY ATTRACTIONS

The south end of the greenway runs adjacent to Northpoint Mall, a regional shopping center with the standard mix of stores. For something different, enjoy a movie midhike (and avoid the hassles of parking your car). As you climb the concrete steps to return to the greenway, turn right and walk down to the end of the trail. On the right is AMC Mansell 14 Crossing Movie Theater; phone (770) 992-9663.

33 BOWMAN'S ISLAND TRAIL

KEY AT-A-GLANCE INFORMATION

LENGTH: 2.9 miles

CONFIGURATION: Double loop

DIFFICULTY: Easy

SCENERY: Some winter views of the Chattahoochee River

EXPOSURE: Full sun at start, then mostly shaded

TRAFFIC: Low

TRAIL SURFACE: Mostly old gravel roads connected by compacted dirt

HIKING TIME: 1.5 hours

ACCESS: Open year-round

MAPS: There is a map at the kiosk at the trailhead, USGS Buford Dam

FACILITIES: Restrooms and picnicking nearby

SPECIAL COMMENTS: Dogs are not allowed to cross into the Bowman Island Unit of the Chattahoochee River National Recreation Area, nor are they allowed in Buford Dam Park. This hike never crosses on to Bowman's Island.

UTM Trailhead Coordinates

UTM Zone (NAD27) 16S

Easting 0769157

Northing 3783386

IN BRIEF

This double-loop trail in the Bowman Island Unit of the Chattahoochee River National Recreation Area circles just below the crest of two hills south of the Buford Dam. Horseback riding is allowed, but this section of the trail is only lightly used.

DESCRIPTION

At the south end of the first parking lot, a modular bridge has been placed over Haw Creek (or McClain's Branch). After crossing the creek, the pathway bears right, crossing a wide, level field that was once a part of the Chattahoochee River floodplain. At 0.1 mile a second path heads off to the right, almost doubling back on the trail as it begins an easy-to-moderate climb to an old road that circles the top of a low hill. Once on this road, there is some elevation change as the pathway climbs and falls, in and out of coves. Much of the pine cover has fallen prey to the pine borer, but there are still some good stands of longleaf. You can see a few homes behind trees, but for the most part they are not obtrusive.

Directions

Take GA 400 north to Exit 14, Buford/Cumming. The exit ramp passes under the overpass, then loops around. Turn right and travel 0.3 miles to GA 9. Turn right (at Burger King and Wachovia) and travel 0.9 miles to Buford Dam Road. Turn right at the Shell station. Drive 4.8 miles, until Buford Dam Road makes a 90-degree left-hand turn; you'll see a wide driveway straight ahead. As you enter the apron, a sign for Lower Pool Park is almost straight ahead. Continue on this dirt road 0.2 miles to the first parking lot on the right. The trailhead is on the north end of the lot.

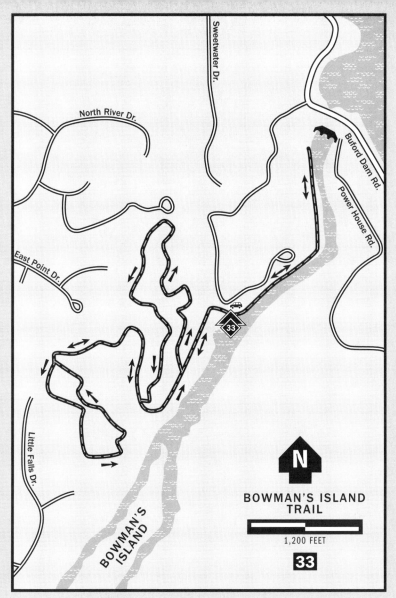

North River Dr.

Sweetwater Dr.

Buford Dam Rd.

Power House Rd.

East Point Dr.

Little Falls Dr.

BOWMAN'S ISLAND

N

BOWMAN'S ISLAND
TRAIL

1,200 FEET

33

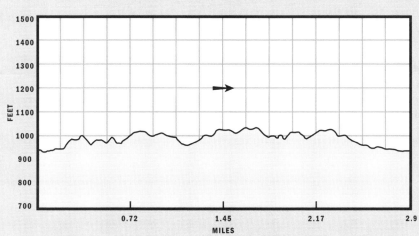

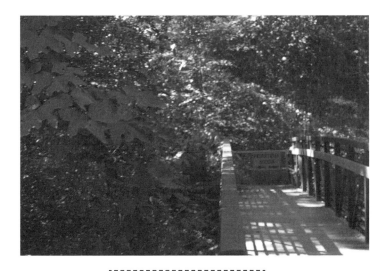

Bridge to Bowman's Island Unit

At the three-way intersection at 0.8 miles, take the pathway that bears left and climbs to the top of the ridge. From here the path drops rapidly but not steeply, finally curving hard to the right and dropping to a wide road 0.3 miles later. Continue straight, following the gravel road as it climbs to another three-way intersection 0.1 mile ahead. The trail turns left, leaving the first loop and joining the second loop 0.3 miles later. Turn left and cross a shallow creek on a wooden bridge 1.5 miles into the hike. Dammed downstream, the river forms a small lake to the left of the path. You can also see homes ahead and on the right.

As the trail follows an old road through a mostly hardwood forest, watch for the occasionally large beech trees throughout the hike. The barrage of oak trees, including red, white, and pin oak, and an occasional maple tree, is typical of a Georgia piedmont forest. The trail drops, and off to the right you can hear the rush of water. In some places you can spot the wide Chattahoochee River, especially in the winter. As the trail circles to the left, it moves away from the river and climbs back to the intersection with the trail from the first loop. Turn right, then make another right and follow the road back to the parking lot.

After crossing the bridge at the start of the trail, turn right and follow the creek to the Chattahoochee River. As the trail turns left at the riverbank, you can usually see the shoals in center; there are frequently waterfowl on or near them, even if a trout fisherman is nearby. Follow the trail to the left, past a "blooper" that warns of an imminent release from Buford Dam. Continue on, moving slightly inland and crossing a boat ramp and picnic area to a prefabricated bridge over the powerhouse channel. Part of the powerhouse is visible from the left side of the bridge. Turn around and retrace your steps to the parking lot.

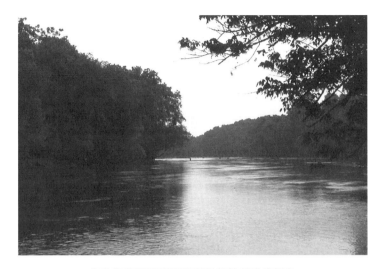

Chattahoochee River at Bowman's Island

NEARBY ATTRACTIONS

The visitor center at the Buford Dam Office provides information on the creation of the dam, facts about Lake Lanier, and a general history of the area around the lake. It is open daily, 8 a.m. to 4:30 p.m. Call (770) 945-9531 for more information.

34 COOK'S TRAIL

KEY AT-A-GLANCE INFORMATION

LENGTH: 8.4 miles

CONFIGURATION: Out-and-back

DIFFICULTY: Easy

SCENERY: Creekside views of Sandy Creek, wetlands, and small lakes

EXPOSURE: Partial shade

TRAFFIC: Moderate

TRAIL SURFACE: Moist dirt that is heavily rooted at times

HIKING TIME: 4.5 hours

ACCESS: Open year-round, dawn–dusk

MAPS: Available at Sandy Creek Nature Center; Sandy Creek Park; USGS Athens East, Athens West, Nicholson, Hull

FACILITIES: Restrooms at either end of the trail

SPECIAL COMMENTS: Cook's Trail can be combined with Lake Chapman Trail (page 176) to create a 13-mile round-trip hike.

UTM Trailhead Coordinates

UTM Zone (NAD27) 17S

Easting   0280664

Northing   3767302

IN BRIEF

Cook's Trail follows the floodplain of Sandy Creek from Lake Chapman in Sandy Creek Park to Sandy Creek Nature Center.

DESCRIPTION

Conceived and developed by Professor Walter L. Cook Jr. of the University of Georgia Forestry and Recreation and Leisure Services, Cook's Trail is an extension of the North Oconee River Greenway, a 3-mile-long paved park that connects Sandy Creek Nature Center to the University of Georgia at Athens on the south and Lake Chapman Trail on the north. The trail follows Sandy Creek from Sandy Creek Park to Sandy Creek Nature Center, which Cook also founded.

The development of Cook's Trail actually began about the time work was being completed on Lake Chapman in the early 1970s when the U.S. Soil Conservation Service wanted to channelize Sandy Creek to control erosion. Professor Charles Aguar led the battle to preserve the natural setting. Cook pushed

---

Directions

Take I-85 North to Exit 106, GA 316, then drive 39.5 miles until you see a sign that says GA 316 ends. Follow the signs for 10 Loop North and take it 4.6 miles to Exit 12, US 441 North/ GA 15/Dr. MLK Pkwy./Commerce. At the end of the ramp, turn left and travel 2.1 miles to Bob Homan Road. Turn right and proceed 0.7 miles, then turn right into Sandy Creek Park. At the pay booth/information kiosk, ask for the map to Cook's Trail. Continue 0.1 mile, turning right at a stop sign. This road curves back to the left, and Campsite Drive heads off to the right. Cross the dam and park in the first parking area.

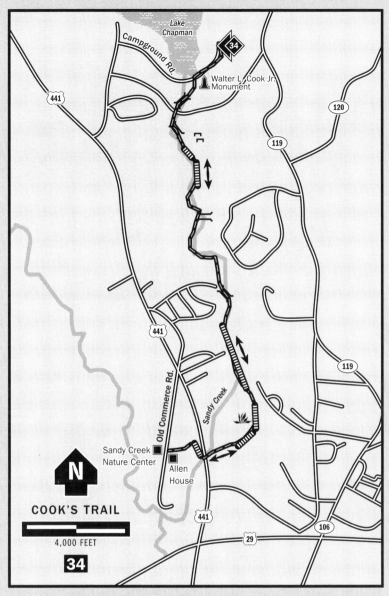

Lake Chapman

Campground Rd.

34

Walter L. Cook Jr. Monument

441

120

119

119

441

Sandy Creek

Old Commerce Rd.

Sandy Creek Nature Center

Allen House

N

COOK'S TRAIL

4,000 FEET

34

441

29

106

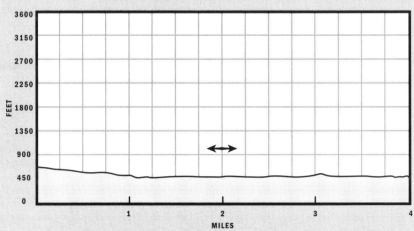

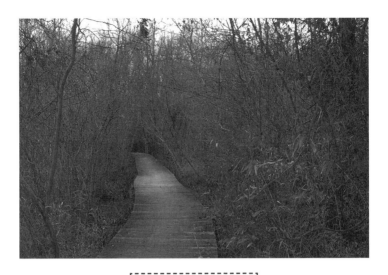

Boardwalk on Cook's Trail

the concept of a nature center not only to preserve the area near the confluence of Sandy Creek and the Oconee River but to educate people as to the importance of forests and their inhabitants in the cycle of life. Following the completion of the nature center, Cook proposed a greenway to connect it to Lake Chapman. Once the land was purchased, Cook personally designed the trail and was lead volunteer of the group that built it.

The trailhead, on the east side of the parking lot, has an information kiosk and a three-page welcome stand that contains a map, an overview of the trail, and trail-use guidelines. As you descend through a loblolly-and-shortleaf-pine forest, a green chain-link fence at 0.2 miles marks the start of the greenway. Cook's Trail continues an easy-to-moderate descent to a three-way trail intersection at 0.4 miles, where a trail provides access to Sandy Creek Park's Lake Chapman Trail (page 176). Turn left and continue the descent into the Sandy Creek river valley. As the descent moderates, the trail begins a long, slow curve to the left. There is a monument to Walter L. Cook Jr. commemorating the effort that he put into the trail. Additionally, there is a good "above it all" view of Sandy Creek, which lies in a valley on the right. About 0.6 miles into the hike, the trail joins the creek, occasionally running along its banks. From this point on, the hike is on a trail that is mostly level, frequently moist (wet after a rain), and heavily rooted. Until the end of the hike, the trail is never more than 100 feet from the creek.

Through a diverse hardwood forest composed mostly of white and post oak and some maple, the trail enters a cleared gas-pipeline field, then crosses the first bridge, at 0.8 miles. When Cook's Trail reaches a tributary of the creek, it normally turns left, heads a few feet inland, crosses the bridge, and then returns to the riverbank. After crossing another tributary and a couple of wetlands, the trail turns left, then makes a right across its first major bridge, with wooden slats and iron railings, at 1.2 miles. This clear creek with high water volume is one of the larger tributaries on the hike. After crossing the bridge, the trail turns right and then left as it rejoins the river. Less than 0.3 miles later is a similar bridge, this time crossing Sandy Creek to an island then crossing Sandy Creek to the far riverbank. Now Sandy Creek is on your left, and the trail gradually climbs.

An intrusive green-roofed home comes into view as the treadway curves to the left at 1.8 miles. One issue that Cook sees with the greenway is that not enough land was purchased, which means development can encroach on the hike's serene beauty. A forested wetland on the right contrasts with the house's backyard on the left, across the creek. Following the forested wetlands is an oxbow lake, created by the ever-changing creek. Once this was a curve in the river, but it was eventually bypassed as the river straightened and the oxbow lake became part of the floodplain. When Sandy Creek runs high, the oxbow lake is flooded and helps keep too much sediment from flowing downstream.

Not very far after you pass a trail on the right, the path turns and crosses Sandy Creek again, quickly entering a heavily rooted, muddy area. Just after 2.6 miles, the path begins to run on a long, elevated walkway as the creek spreads out to form a wetland. The segments of boardwalk are interspersed with short sections of normally moist, rooted, occasionally muddy track. Once again, houses intrude on pristine nature. We flushed a red-shouldered hawk from its perch.

Over the next 0.6 miles, the trail circles a large wetland area to the east and south of Sandy Creek before rejoining a wider, fuller creek at 3.6 miles. Shortly after rejoining the river, the pathway turns right, crosses a wooden-planked iron bridge, then turns left at the far side of the creek and passes under US 441. After exiting the bridge, the treadway parallels the road, heading north until the signed entrance to Sandy Creek Nature Center, at 3.9 miles. The trail makes a sweeping curve to the left, joining Pine Ridge Trail after the marked Screech Owl Trail leaves only to quickly rejoin Cooks Trail. Turn right and follow the trail to the Allen house (circa 1900), which is at the nature center trailhead. After visiting the area, retrace your route back to the car.

NEARBY ATTRACTIONS

Sandy Creek Nature Center has the ENSAT (Environment, Natural Science, and Appropriate Technology) Center, a regionally focused environmental education center that demonstrates how to incorporate modern technological advances into construction projects to reduce their impact on the environment. Two exhibits within the museum highlight the Coastal Community and the Wetlands Community, including life-cycle information on endangered loggerhead turtles and a 1,500-gallon aquarium and 500-gallon feeding tank. The center also has miles of hiking trails and is the northern end of the North Oconee Greenway, a concrete-paved multiuse trail that connects to the University of Georgia trail system.

35 DESOTO FALLS TRAIL

KEY AT-A-GLANCE INFORMATION

LENGTH: 2.3 miles

CONFIGURATION: Double out-and-back trails

DIFFICULTY: Easy, except for the climb to the Lower Falls, which is easy–moderate

SCENERY: Mountain streams, 2 waterfalls

EXPOSURE: Full shade

TRAFFIC: Moderate

TRAIL SURFACE: Compacted soil, dirt road

HIKING TIME: 1.25 hours

ACCESS: Hiking trail is open year-round, 7 a.m.–10 p.m.

MAPS: USGS Neel's Gap

FACILITIES: Restrooms, picnic tables with grills; camping from early May–November

SPECIAL COMMENTS: Many of the unusual names in this area are Cherokee in origin. In 1838 the Cherokee were forcibly removed by the State of Georgia in a tragedy known as the Trail of Tears. Only their names for places serve to remember them.

UTM Trailhead Coordinates

UTM Zone (NAD27) 17S

Easting   0233011

Northing 3844138

IN BRIEF

This is a wonderful waterfalls walk with a nearby babbling brook in the north Georgia mountains. Plan on spending the whole day doing your choice of the multiple short hikes listed in the Nearby Attractions.

DESCRIPTION

Hernando Desoto explored Georgia in 1540 and 1541, ranging from the extreme southwest corner near Bainbridge to Augusta, and over to the northwest, in search of gold. In the 1880s a Spanish breastplate was found near the falls, giving Desoto Falls its name and lasting legacy. Many scholars did not think finding a breastplate intact more than 300 years later was possible until a 1540s-era Spanish sword was discovered intact near Rome, Georgia, in 1983.

At the entrance to the trail's parking lot is a brown-roofed trailhead kiosk where you pay the $2 National Park Service fee. The pathway, to the left of the kiosk, is covered with pea-sized gravel and curves left as it falls to a picnic area within the park. As the trail levels, it turns right and runs along Frogtown Creek.

Directions

Take GA 400 to the end. Turn left on US 19/GA 60. There is a Shell station, Waffle House, and Home Depot at this intersection. Continue 4.1 miles, then turn right on US 19/GA 60/GA 9. Drive 8.2 miles, until GA 60 goes straight at US 19/GA 9; curve around to the right at Stonepile Gap. Continue on this road for another 5.3 miles to Turner's Corner. Turn left on US 19/129 and travel 5.3 miles to Desoto Falls, on the left. Parking is in the first lot on the left; walk to the trailhead kiosk next to the restrooms.

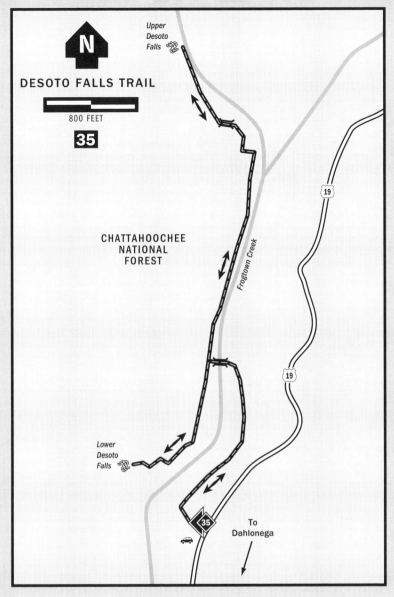

DESOTO FALLS TRAIL

Upper
Desoto
Falls

800 FEET

35

CHATTAHOOCHEE
NATIONAL
FOREST

Frogtown Creek

19

19

Lower
Desoto
Falls

35

To
Dahlonega

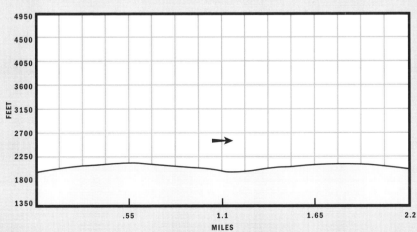

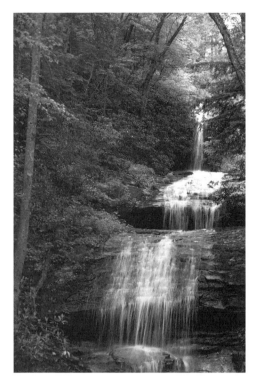

Frogtown was the settlers' name for a Cherokee village near the creek. According to Cherokee mythology, a great frog, Walesi, lived in the gap above the creek. The village was called Walesi-yi or "Place of the Great Frog." In 1946 the Appalachian Trail Conference changed the name of Frogtown Gap to Neel's Gap. Only the stone building at the top of the mountain, Walesi-yi, honors the Cherokee by preserving their name for the area.

After you turn left on an asphalt road, you'll see a path off to the left, just past the camp host's site, crossing Frogtown Creek on a wooden bridge. A sign on the far side of the bridge tells the story of Desoto Falls. Turn left, and follow the path along Frogtown Creek before making a hard right as it begins an easy-to-moderate switchback climb to the Lower Falls. Just past a large rock outcrop, the path turns right, rising to a viewing platform directly in front of the 35-foot-tall Lower Falls. Typical of a north Georgia waterfall, the water drops off a ledge and cascades a few feet to a second ledge, where it freefalls to a second cascade, then to a third ledge-cascade combination. After visiting for a few minutes, retrace your steps to the bridge over Frogtown Creek.

As you pass the sign at the bridge, the footpath enters a wide, level floodplain of the river in a diverse pine and hardwood forest typical of the north Georgia mountains. The canopy of trees contains white and chestnut oak, loblolly pine, tulip poplar, and sweetgum. Occasionally, hickory, red oak, and pin oak can be found. After reaching the confluence of Frogtown Creek and an unnamed tributary, the footpath climbs and descends three short hills near the creek. After you cross a wooden bridge, you'll find a notice informing you that the trail to Upper Desoto Falls is closed for now. Beginning in 1993 with a snowstorm commonly called "the Storm of the Century," and followed by 1994's Palm Sunday killer tornadoes and Hurricane Juan in 1995, the north Georgia mountains were repeatedly raked by damaging storms. Downed trees make ascending to the Upper Falls very difficult, but don't worry—the middle falls are spectacular.

Turn left and climb to the viewing platform. Coming off of Blood Mountain, a narrow stream of water drops to a ledge where the stream widens as it cascades down to a second ledge. From here the falls make a brief drop to a third shelf that juts out over a large rock. At the bottom of the falls, a small pool with a number of larger rocks makes for a scenic picture. If you want to get good photos, plan to be here in the morning of the first sunny day after a rain, when the falls are at their fullest.

NEARBY ATTRACTIONS

Turn left out of the park and climb Blood Mountain to Neel's Gap. On the right is Mountain Crossings at Walesi-yi, a stone lodge built by the CCC in 1938 that now houses a hiking equipment shop that's worth the stop. Turn right out of Walesi-yi and travel 0.25 miles to the Byron Herbert Reece Memorial Trail parking lot on the left. This access trail steeply climbs to the A.T. on Blood Mountain. Farther down the mountain is Vogel State Park, with Bear Hair Trail (5 miles) and Coosa Bald Trail (11 miles), plus camping and cabins. Watch for Spillway Falls on the left, after the entrance. Turn left on GA 180, climbing to Sosebee Cove. This 0.3-mile hike is great between mid-April and late September, when wildflowers are in bloom.

Farther down on GA 180, Lake Winfield Scott, on the left, has additional A.T. access. In Suches, turn left on GA 60. After passing through Woody Gap, the road descends to Stonepile Gap. Go straight ahead to Dahlonega on US 19. This small town was the center of America's first gold rush. The State of Georgia established a gold museum in the old county courthouse in 1965. Smith House, one of the best family-style restaurants in the Southeast, is one block south of the museum and worth a visit. Hours vary; for details, see its Web site at **www.smithhouse.com** or call (706) 867-7000 or (800) 852-9577.

36 EAST AND WEST LAKE TRAILS

KEY AT-A-GLANCE INFORMATION

LENGTH: 5.4 miles

CONFIGURATION: Loop

DIFFICULTY: Moderate

SCENERY: This loop circles Chicopee Lake, on the south end of Chicopee Woods Nature Preserve, affording both long-distance and lakeshore views. There are some creekside views along both the East and West Lake Trails.

EXPOSURE: Full sun in the area around Chicopee Lake, mostly shaded along the rest of the trail

TRAFFIC: Light, except in the vicinity of the lake, where traffic is moderate

TRAIL SURFACE: Gravel road, compacted soil, cement in the interpreted area of the lakeshore

HIKING TIME: 3 hours

ACCESS: Open year-round

MAPS: Trail map available at Elachee Center; USGS Chestnut Mountain

FACILITIES: Restrooms available Monday–Saturday at Elachee Center and Chicopee Lake

SPECIAL COMMENTS: There is plenty of wildlife to see throughout the hike.

UTM Trailhead Coordinates

UTM Zone (NAD27) 17S

Easting 0239065

Northing 3792623

IN BRIEF

This loop trail explores the foothills of the Blue Ridge Mountains through a typical hardwood forest from the Elachee Nature Science Center to the Chicopee Aquatic Studies Center at Chicopee Lake.

DESCRIPTION

Following a developed dirt road (notice the runoff ditches on either side) that ascends 0.1 mile, the trail then begins to descend at an easy-to-moderate pace over the next 0.3 miles. After a four-way intersection at the top of the hill, the road becomes very rocky. Tree limbs cover the road as it bears left at 0.4 miles, while the trail bears right and enters the woods. Briefly, the orange-blazed trail becomes loamy and is covered by sand. As you begin walking downhill along a low ridge, the forest is mostly made up of post and white oak, American beech, and native dogwood. Crossing a wooden bridge over a normally dry gully at 0.5 miles, the trail quickly traverses a second bridge, just after a large post oak.

Directions

Take I-85 North to Exit 113 (GA 365/I-985/ Lanier Parkway), then take I-985 North to Exit 16 (GA 53/Oakwood/Dawsonville). At end of the ramp, get in the right-hand left-turn lane. Turn at the light, then go under the bridge and carefully merge right into the "keep moving" lane for southbound traffic. At 0.3 miles turn right at the first traffic light and travel 0.7 miles. Turn left onto GA 13 at the traffic light. Drive 1.6 miles and make two hard right-hand turns into Chicopee Woods. In 1 mile you'll see trailhead parking straight ahead, just across a bridge over I-985. Walk to a brown kiosk at the east end of the parking lot.

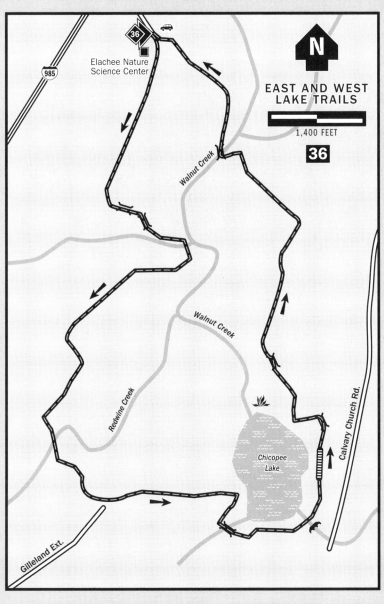

EAST AND WEST
LAKE TRAILS

1,400 FEET

36

Elachee Nature
Science Center

Walnut Creek

Walnut Creek

Redwine Creek

Chicopee
Lake

Calvary Church Rd.

Gilleland Ext.

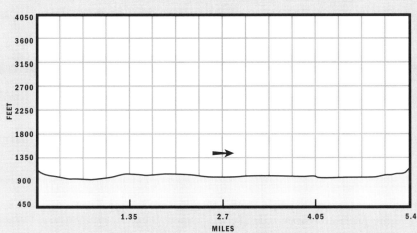

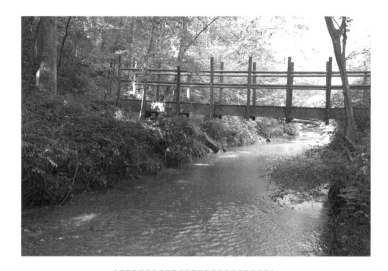

Bridge over Vulture Rock Creek

After the second bridge, the trail narrows and follows the riverbank down-hill through an old-growth forest. After climbing away from the riverbank, the trail begins a rapid switchback descent until it bears right and descends stairs. At this point, West Lake Trail turns left, joining Dunlop Trail along a wide, well-defined river on your right. Side trails lead down to and cross the river, but you should continue along the riverbank until you come to a wooden bridge. Cross the bridge; on the far side, the trail reaches a T-intersection. Turn left.

West Lake Trail briefly follows the river and then makes a hard right turn and climbs a rooted, occasionally rocky pathway through a second-growth forest. As you move away from the river, the number of ferns quickly decreases; as you climb, the number of pines increases. At 1.1 miles the trail joins an old road, soon making a hard right turn to leave this road. Now the trail begins a zigzag climb, joining another road about halfway up the hill. At the top of the hill, the trail turns left at a map stand (which has no map). There is a small, hand-painted sign that says "1.4 miles," the distance to Chicopee Lake.

Falling to a dry creek at just under 2 miles, West Lake Trail crosses the creek, turns left, then curves back around as it begins to climb. A bridge is scheduled to be built here in the near future. Making a moderate-to-difficult climb up a steep-sided hill, the footpath turns left at another hand-painted sign and begins a some-what easier descent to the first view of Chicopee Lake, at 2.8 miles. Make a note of the kiosk to your right, then explore the several good viewing areas.

The lake is a diverse ecosystem that attracts a wide variety of animals. When we were there, a snowy egret busied itself searching for food in the marshy wet-lands where the lake forms, while a family of otters churned the water along the distant lakeshore. Geese landed in the lake, taking a rest on their long journey south. Above, a red-tailed hawk soared on the thermals, perhaps looking for food, perhaps just enjoying the ride.

Return to the kiosk, and with it on your right, walk straight ahead, as if you had made a hard right turn from the trail coming in to the viewing area. A brown sign quickly confirms that you are on West Lake Trail. Over the next mile, the trail circles the lake, moving inland and up to a boardwalk crossing a small wetlands and stream before returning lakeside and heading down to the lakeshore and a popular fishing area. Follow the trail to the right, climbing and circling to the left before coming down the steps into full sun as you walk across the top of the dam that impounds Walnut Creek to form Chicopee Lake.

From the dam there are scenic views of the lake to the left and Walnut Creek to the right. At a mailbox the trail bears slightly left, toward a white building with bathrooms and interpretive information. Walk around the building, turn right, and walk toward a white fence near a main road. An interpretive sign describes the flowers in the dry meadow before you. Turn around, keeping the parking lot on your right, to follow the sidewalk to a cement path on the left down to the boardwalk-style dock on the lake. This area is also signed and indicates that the lake is home to both osprey and bald eagles in addition to a wide variety of smaller animals, waterfowl, and fish.

Return to the parking lot and make a left turn on the sidewalk. Continue to an unmarked but well-worn path to the left, just before the ranger's cottage, and head into a forest of red maple and white oak also sporting varieties of pine. Fully shaded and now called East Lake Trail, it joins Cavalry Creek at 3.6 miles, soon making a hard left-hand turn into the creek and up the bank on the other side. The trail crosses creeks three times over the next 0.2 miles, then climbs a hill. Near the top, at 3.9 miles, the trail turns right and joins an old road before quickly turning left to leave the roadbed.

East Lake Trail makes an easy descent to a bridge over a boulder-strewn creek. After the bridge, the trail turns left and briefly levels off before beginning an extended climb to a hilltop. Difficult at first, the climb moderates as it rises, becoming easy near the top. A pine blowdown caused by the southern pine beetle extends over the next 0.7 miles. At a kiosk near the top of the hill, East Lake Trail joins Dunlap Trail and bears right.

Coming to the top of a hill at 4.6 miles, the combined Dunlap and East Lake Trail make a hard left, although an unmarked path continues straight ahead. Now falling at a moderate-to-difficult grade over the next 0.2 miles, the pathway makes another hard left as it starts to run adjacent to a wetland near Walnut Creek. After crossing a bridge, the trail turns right and combines switchbacks and stairs to quickly ascend from the river valley. East Lake Trail ends at a T-intersection with Mathis Loop Trail. Turn left on Mathis Loop to return to your car.

Mathis Loop is well marked. At Walnut Creek Trail, Mathis Loop turns right, then bears right at a small rain shelter. Just over 0.1 mile after the shelter, a short trail on the left returns you to the trailhead.

37 HARD LABOR CREEK TRAIL

KEY AT-A-GLANCE INFORMATION

LENGTH: 2.1 miles

CONFIGURATION: Double loop, almost a figure 8

DIFFICULTY: Moderate

SCENERY: Cascades, deep ravines, long-distance view of small lake

EXPOSURE: Generally shaded

TRAFFIC: Light

TRAIL SURFACE: Compacted dirt that becomes rocky and heavily rooted at times

HIKING TIME: 1.5 hours

ACCESS: Tuesday–Sunday, 7 a.m.–10 p.m.

MAPS: Available at Trading Post; USGS Rutledge North

FACILITIES: Restrooms at trailhead, picnic tables nearby

SPECIAL COMMENTS: Lake Brantley is only occasionally visible from the trail.

IN BRIEF

Composed of Lake Brantley Nature Trail and Beaver Pond Trail, Hard Labor Creek Hiking Trail follows various creeks and explores ridges within Hard Labor Creek State Park.

DESCRIPTION

This is one of the most unusually named Georgia State Parks, and park rangers are often asked, "Where did the name 'Hard Labor' come from?" According to one legend, slaves who had to clear the ground found it so rocky that they called the area "Hard Labor." Another legend has Native Americans naming the creek for the difficulty of crossing it in wet weather. The CCC had both a camp and a rock quarry in the park.

To get to the trailhead from the parking area, walk back toward the trading post,

UTM Trailhead Coordinates

UTM Zone (NAD27)   17S

Easting   0258360

Northing   3727853

Directions

From Atlanta take I-20 East to Exit 105, Rutledge/Newborn Road. At the end of the ramp, turn left. Go 0.3 miles to a four-way stop at Davis Academy Road. Continue straight. There is a second four-way stop at Rutledge Grocery (US 278/GA 12), at 2.3 miles. Continue straight, until Newborn Road ends at Dixie Highway, at 2.6 miles. Turn left. Note that traffic to the right has no stop. Go 1 block and turn right, onto Fairplay Road. At West Main Street (the center of historic Rutledge) there is a four-way stop on weekends. Continue straight 1.3 miles. Fairplay Road bears left and continues to the park entrance 0.9 miles ahead. At 0.5 miles after the entrance, turn left on Knox Chapel Road. Turn right 0.4 miles later, onto an unnamed road that leads to the Trading Post). Pay the $3 fee here or at one of the green self-help fee stations. Once past the trading post, turn left into one of the diagonal parking spaces on the other side.

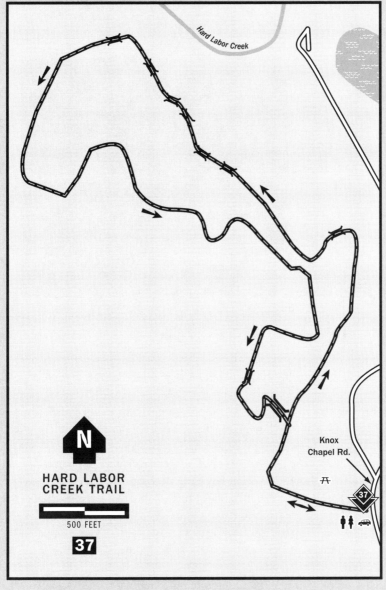

Hard Labor Creek

Knox
Chapel Rd.

N

HARD LABOR
CREEK TRAIL

500 FEET

37

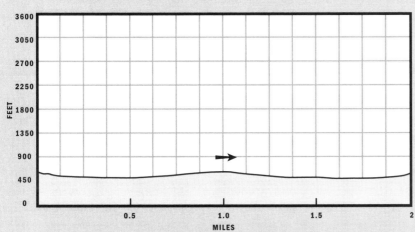

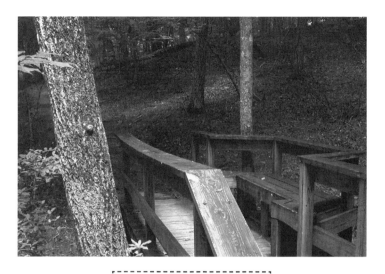

Clever bench and bridge design

turning right onto the road that leads to the comfort station. Hard Labor Creek Trail is on the left, in the woods behind an open picnic area. A brown pole with trail names and distances marks the start of the trail. Two loop trails, Lake Brantley Nature Trail and Beaver Dam Trail, make up Hard Labor Creek Trail.

Beginning on the yellow-blazed Lake Brantley Nature Trail, the hike leads through a typical Georgia piedmont pine forest. Leaves and pine needles cover the relatively level ground that was once home to antebellum plantations. Shortly after the start of the hike, the trail begins to descend and curves to the right.

Interpretive Ranger Amanda Westbrook, who regularly teaches classes on trail safety and plant identification, told us of the native azaleas that bloom in the early spring along the path. She also made sure we used an insect repellent because of the large number of ticks on these trails. For more information on ticks and other insects, see the Introduction, page 9.

At 0.1 mile the trail climbs a granite outcropping, then descends over rocks and roots to a wood-and-dirt stairway leading deep into a ravine. Completely shaded, the path has a wooden rail on the left. Large gopher holes and a downed tree make this area somewhat difficult to navigate. At 0.2 miles the trail splits at two wooden bridges. Take the bridge directly in front of you.

As you cross the bridge, look to the right at a large ravine being created by a tributary. Shortly after the bridge, there is a tree carved by woodpeckers and termites; walk around it. Next, a path to the right leads to a campground, which you can see is just behind a stand of trees. Falling to the creek bed the trail levels and becomes heavily rooted.

At 0.4 miles there is another wooden bridge built by the Young Adult Conservation Corps (YACC). Conceived during the Carter administration and loosely based on the CCC, this program provided employment to disadvantaged kids in the late 1970s, putting them to work on public land projects throughout the United States. After the bridge the trail climbs to the start of the red-blazed Beaver Dam Trail, which heads off to the right and splits shortly after the turn. Take the trail straight ahead.

As you descend toward a creek bed, notice how the size of the trees starts to increase. Some of the trees measure 12 to 13 feet around, indicating this is an older-growth forest. A wooden bridge at 0.6 miles is partially damaged, probably from one of the fallen pines in the area. After navigating around the bridge damage and the pine graveyard (caused by rampant pine-beetle infestation), Beaver Dam Trail climbs to the middle of a low ridge. Soon the path falls to a wooden bridge over a deep gully. After descending a few stairs at the end of the bridge, the path bears right. Two more bridges follow in rapid succession, and then the path falls to the wide, level plain of the creek, which it follows briefly.

As Beaver Dam Trail turns left at 0.8 miles, it begins to climb alongside another stream and takes on a different personality. Now rocky and heavily rooted, the path climbs along a creek that cascades in spots. Finally, just short of a mile into the journey, the footpath leaves the stream, enters heavily shaded forest, and begins to climb to a ridgetop covered with maple, oak, and beech trees.

From the ridge the trail begins to switchback, sometimes descending steeply back to the start of the loop. As you reach the short return path to Lake Brantley Trail, turn right. You'll take just a few steps before the red blazes of Beaver Dam Trail are almost seamlessly replaced by the yellow blazes of Lake Brantley Trail. At the intersection, Lake Brantley Trail bears right, then, a few steps up the trail, it begins to make a harder right-hand turn.

The trail begins a moderate climb through a partially sunny hardwood forest as you double back to the trailhead on the other side of the valley. From this peak the footpath begins to descend into the basin toward the start of the loop. At 1.8 miles Lake Brantley Trail crosses the longest bridge of the hike, returning to the start of the loop trail. Turn right to return to the trailhead.

NEARBY ATTRACTIONS

Historic Madison, Georgia, (www.madisonga.org) is the town that General Sherman didn't burn. For more information call (800) 709-7406 or visit the Welcome Center on Jefferson Street, Monday through Friday, 8:30 a.m. to 5 p.m.; Saturday, 10 a.m. to 5 p.m.; and Sunday, 1 p.m. to 4 p.m.

38 JONES BRIDGE TRAIL

KEY AT-A-GLANCE INFORMATION

LENGTH: 5.2 miles

CONFIGURATION: Loop

DIFFICULTY: Easy

SCENERY: Historic bridge, riverside views

EXPOSURE: Full sun in the vicinity of the historic bridge, full shade elsewhere

TRAFFIC: Heavy near the bridge; moderate down to the boat launch; light south of the launch

TRAIL SURFACE: Compacted soil

HIKING TIME: 2 hours

ACCESS: Open year-round, dawn–dusk

MAPS: Available at park headquarters at Island Ford (page 30); USGS Norcross, Duluth, Chamblee

FACILITIES: Restrooms, boat launch, some picnic tables, fishing dock

SPECIAL COMMENTS: Jones Bridge was a privately owned toll bridge that was built in 1904 and ceased operation in 1922. Before that time, a ferry crossed the river at roughly the same spot.

UTM Trailhead Coordinates

UTM Zone (NAD27) 16S

Easting   0754964

Northing 3765484

IN BRIEF

This hike explores Jones Bridge, climbing into nearby hills that allow long-distance views of some of Atlanta's most expensive homes and then following the floodplain of the Chatta-hoochee, climbing to explore a ridge and returning to loop around a second floodplain.

DESCRIPTION

Ferries were the first privately owned businesses to span Georgia's mighty rivers. With increased competition from railroads, ferry owners began to build bridges and charge a toll for crossing. As the government began building roads in the 1920s, many of the old bridges quickly became obsolete. Jones Bridge's usefulness (in the mind of its owner) came to an end in the early 1920s, when it was abandoned, although farmers did continue to use it until the wooden planking rotted. In 1940 World War II sent scrap metal prices soaring, even though the United States had not entered the war yet. A group of workmen began dismantling the southern end of Jones Bridge, working in plain sight one day. People didn't

Directions

Take GA 400 North to Holcomb Bridge Road/140 East. Turn right at the end of the ramp. Travel 4.2 miles to Barnwell Road (there's a CVS and a SunTrust on the corner). Ignore the first brown sign, which is the entrance to the Environmental Center. At 1.6 miles turn right at the Jones Bridge Unit sign. Follow the road as it curves around and switches back, passing a small parking lot on the right for cars with fishing boats. At 1.2 miles the main parking lot opens up. Turn left, park, and return to the trailhead kiosk on the south end of the parking lot.

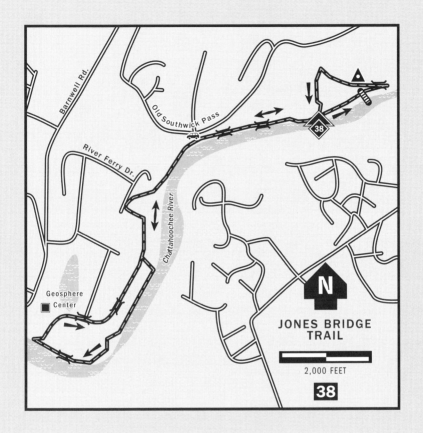

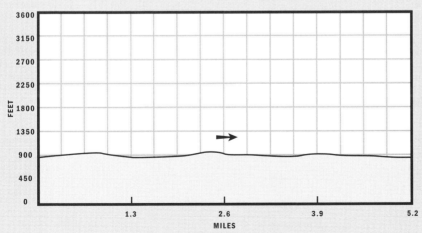

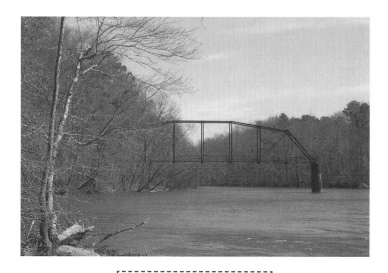

Remaining half of Jones Bridge

ask any questions until the men didn't show up the second day. Then folks realize the workers had made off with the scrap metal, probably selling it a piece at a time so that their theft would go undetected in the lucrative Atlanta market.

From the trailhead kiosk, follow a wide dirt road to make an easy descent through a diverse hardwood forest to a four-way intersection 200 feet from the start. Take a minute to walk down to the riverbank, straight ahead, and enjoy the view of the Chattahoochee. On returning, turn right and follow the riverbank, keeping the river on your right. The trail runs some 20 feet inside the bank, and large rock outcroppings tell the river's story. As you pass the outcroppings on the left, take a close look at the water-worn edges and eroded strata in the rock. Before the river was controlled by Buford Dam—20 miles north as the river flows—water levels would fluctuate much more than they do today. The rock, which would be covered only in an unusual circumstance today, routinely flooded before 1953. As you continue along the trail, the floodplain opens up into a park, and a dock for both fishing and viewing extends onto the river, on your right. In the distance the half-span of Jones Bridge waits for another crew to finish the job begun in 1940.

Continue straight ahead toward the bridge past a trail on the left and over a wooden bridge that crosses a stream. Finally, as you approach an intrusive chain-link fence, you'll reach the bridge, which juts out over the Chattahoochee River. Jones Bridge Road, which is still a major road in north Fulton County, ran to this point, crossed the river on the bridge, and continued on the south side of the Chattahoochee. There are a number of large pines in the area. The trail continues a short way along the riverbank, next to the fence.

From the bridge turn around and begin walking the inside of the open field toward a creek crossing and map stand. After the wet-foot crossing, the path joins a road that bears right and begins to climb into the forest. As the trail begins a moderate ascent, it curves away from the riverbank. At 0.8 miles the climb eases as the roadway runs nearly level at the ridgetop. An easy descent returns you to the north end of the parking lot. Continue to the trailhead, but turn right and follow the riverbank, keeping the Chattahoochee on the left. Here the floodplain is wider, not constrained by the hills adjacent to the river. We flushed a blue heron at the first bridge, just after the turn.

Crossing another wooden bridge at 1.3 miles, the pathway takes you to a third bridge and the fishing ramp parking area 0.3 miles later. Walk straight across the lot, and the path continues, almost immediately crossing another bridge. Turning inland at 1.8 miles at a flight of wooden steps, the trail begins another moderate climb into the Chattahoochee River watershed, dropping to a gravel road, and then climbing again. Notice the American beech trees at the top of the mountain some 0.2 miles after the start of the climb. There are four or five massive beech trees, and much smaller ones in the nearby forest. As the pathway begins to descend, you'll see a home on the left, between the trail and the river.

Come to a three-way intersection with a map stand at 2.3 miles, turn left, and continue an easy descent toward the river, coming to a second intersection a couple hundred feet later. Take the trail on the right, which runs fairly level down to a wooden bridge at 2.6 miles. The footpath curves gently right, and a crossover trail heads off to the left. Just past the crossover trail is an intersection, where the trail bears left; next, you come to a bridge as you enter an open field near the Geosphere Center. At a grassy road leading to the center, turn left; the trail begins an easy descent, curving right at a map stand at 3 miles, then making a hard left less than 0.1 mile later.

After following the riverbank another 0.1 mile, the footpath curves left, away from the bank, to a right-hand turn at a three-way intersection, crossing a bridge, making another right and then yet another right-hand turn as the trail rejoins the river at 3.2 miles. After passing two side trails on the left, take a few steps up to a low ridge in an area of large trees. As the trail bears left, a trail heads off to the right, then the footpath curves right and another trail comes in from the right. At 3.9 miles the pathway crosscuts a historic road; look for a map stand 100 feet to the left, and follow the trail to it. Turn right and retrace your steps to the car.

39 LAKE CHAPMAN TRAIL

KEY AT-A-GLANCE INFORMATION

LENGTH: 4.6 miles

CONFIGURATION: Out-and-back

DIFFICULTY: Easy

SCENERY: Lake views throughout the hike, and an excellent "above it all" view

EXPOSURE: Mostly shaded

TRAFFIC: Moderate

TRAIL SURFACE: Compacted dirt

HIKING TIME: 2 hours

ACCESS: Open year-round

MAPS: Available at Sandy Creek Park entrance kiosk and office; USGS Nicholson

FACILITIES: Restrooms at trailhead; camping

SPECIAL COMMENTS: This trail can be combined with Cook's Trail (page 156) for a 13-mile round-trip hike from the Sandy Creek Nature Center.

UTM Trailhead Coordinates

UTM Zone (NAD27) 17S

Easting   0280132

Northing 3769317

IN BRIEF

Lake Chapman Trail follows the lakeshore in Sandy Creek Park throughout most of the journey, circling part of the lakeshore and exploring wooded coves in two places. It is a popular fishing lake, and migratory waterfowl are common in spring and fall.

DESCRIPTION

About 260 acres when it's at full pool, picturesque Lake Chapman is actually smaller than it appears in real life, surrounded by 782-acre Sandy Creek Park. Athens-Clarke County Leisure Services Department operates the dam that controls the lake and Sandy Creek Park, which entirely encompasses the lake. According to facilities supervisor Bobby Kerce, Lake Chapman was designed to control floodwaters and sediment flow in the Sandy Creek watershed. Additionally, the lake is designated for recreation and as an emergency water supply for the city of Athens. When the dam was built in the early 1980s, the watershed was not threatened. Today the Sandy Creek watershed faces many challenges, including urban sprawl.

Directions ——————————————————➤

Take I-85 North to Exit 106, GA 316. Drive 39.5 miles on GA 316 until you see a sign that says GA 316 ends. Follow the signs for 10 Loop North and travel 4.6 miles to Exit 12, US 441 North/GA 15/Dr. MLK Pkwy./Commerce. At the end of the ramp, turn left and travel 2.1 miles to Bob Homan Road. Turn right and proceed 0.7 miles, then turn right into Sandy Creek Park. Pay the $2 entrance fee at the kiosk and continue 0.1 mile, turning right at a stop sign. This road curves back to the left, and Campsite Drive heads off to the right. Cross the dam and park in the first parking area.

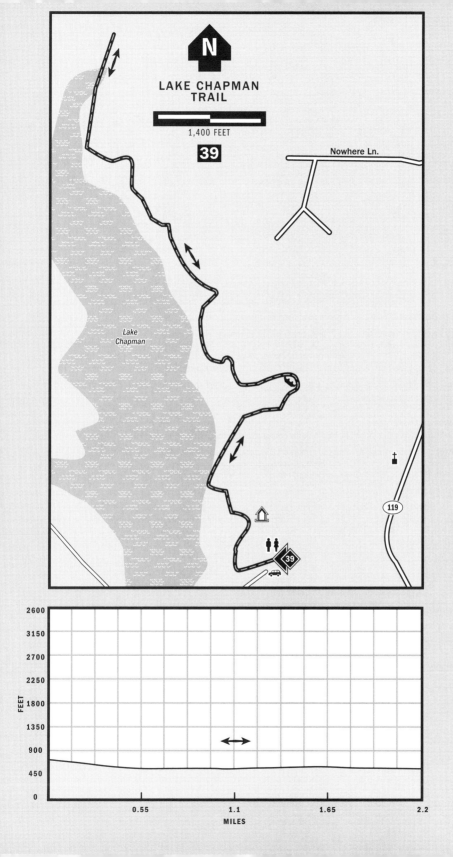

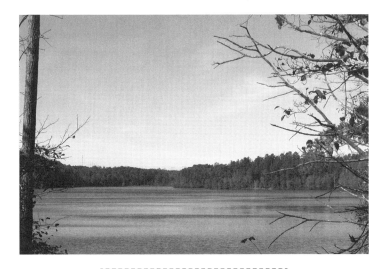

Serene Lake Chapman on Sandy Creek

An urban planner's answer to sprawl is green space like Sandy Creek Park.

Fishing is a popular sport, and according to the Georgia Department of Natural Resources, bream, bass, crappie, and catfish comprise the majority of fish taken from the lake. Only boats with electric motors are permitted, and the Georgia Outdoor Recreation Program regularly holds classes on sailing on the lake. Canoeing is also popular on the flat-water lake. From time to time, Sandy Creek Park employees, on nights with a full moon, take folks for a romantic canoe trip on the lake.

From the parking lot, the trail begins as a paved path to restrooms directly opposite the entrance to Cook's Trail (page 156). When the paved path curves to the right, continue straight ahead to a gravel road and two poles with a chain between them to prevent vehicular traffic. The gravel road begins to curve to the right and it enters a shortleaf pine forest. At the end of the curve, the road splits into two, one continuing the easy curve, the other curving harder to the right. Take the second road, which parallels the lakeshore but does not run adjacent to it. There are wilderness campsites throughout the area.

At 0.2 miles, just past a trail on the left, there is a massive pine blowdown caused by the Southern pine beetle on the right. At the bottom of an easy descent, the trail meets the shoreline for the first time. Both Lake Chapman and the trail begin a sweeping turn right to follow the shore into a cove. This marks the end of the wilderness camping area. Notice that the trees increase in size as you move deeper into this hardwood cove. Watch for sweetgum, winged elm, black walnut, persimmon, and native dogwood in the mostly oak forest. In season the smell of honeysuckle occasionally wafts across the path; Christmas ferns, American beautyberry, and muscadine are easy to spot here.

The normally wide treadway narrows for a wet-foot crossing of a stream at 0.7 miles, then widens again. Just past an earthen dam at 0.8 miles, Buckeye

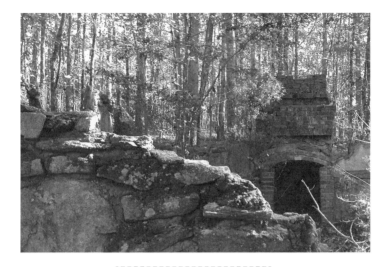

Remains of a 1950's-era cabin

Horse Trail joins Lake Chapman Trail from the right. Shortly, Buckeye Trail exits, also to the right. A little more than a mile into the hike, the horse trail briefly rejoins Lakeside Trail, then heads off to the right again.

Climb 60 feet for an excellent "above it all" view of most of the lake. Large waterfowl are common on the lake, and blue heron can be seen year-round. Park assistant Jessica Banks told us that, in addition to deer, the park has red and gray fox and coyote. The trail begins an easy descent, and the path curves to the right as it enters a small cove of the lake. On the right at 1.3 miles, the stone footers and brick fireplace of a one-room cabin adjoin the trail, remnants of a forestry project from the 1950s that was never completed. Beyond the building is a muddy wet-foot crossing of a tributary of Sandy Creek. Lakeside Trail rejoins the main body of the lake, then curves right, into another cove. Turn left when Lakeside Trail reaches a T-intersection with the horse trail, at 1.5 miles.

As Lakeside Trail rejoins Lake Chapman, it slowly curves to the right, then curves inland as it rises in a brief, easy-to-moderate climb to a rock outcrop at the top of the hill. As the trail descends, a side trail joins the main trail at a 45-degree angle. Take the side trail for excellent views, bearing in mind that the descent is moderate to difficult. On the main path, the moderate descent ends as the path turns right just after the side trail rejoins the main trail. At 1.7 miles there is another long-distance view of the lakeshore.

The trail turns left after a wet-foot crossing, then curves back around to the right as it climbs into a cove that signals the lake's end at a river too deep to ford. Lake Chapman once again becomes Sandy Creek in a forested wetland at the end of the cove. In the future Sandy Creek Park intends to connect the creek and another wetlands on the far side with a bridge. This will join Lakeside Trail with Swimming Deer Trail, creating a loop of almost 6 miles.

40   LAUREL RIDGE TRAIL

KEY AT-A-GLANCE INFORMATION

LENGTH: 3.8 miles

CONFIGURATION: Loop

DIFFICULTY: Moderate, although the climb out of Chattahoochee River Valley is difficult

SCENERY: River views, lakeshore, Buford Dam

EXPOSURE: Mostly shaded

TRAFFIC: Moderate

TRAIL SURFACE: Packed dirt, with cement paths in parks

HIKING TIME: 2.5 hours

ACCESS: Open year-round; may be closed during times of heightened security

MAPS: Interpreted map available at U.S. Army Corps of Engineers visitor center; USGS Buford Dam

FACILITIES: Restrooms in multiple places along trail, water fountains, garbage pails, playgrounds

SPECIAL COMMENTS: No pets allowed on trail

UTM Trailhead Coordinates

UTM Zone (NAD27) 16S

Easting 0770112

Northing 3783401

IN BRIEF

Laurel Ridge Trail explores the bank of the Chattahoochee River, climbs low foothills of the Blue Ridge Mountains, and ventures into coves claimed by Lake Lanier. In the first 0.5 miles of the trail, there are several long-distance views of Buford Dam and Lower Pool Park.

DESCRIPTION

Atlanta's growth created demand for two fundamental commodities—water and electrical power. Starting in 1950, the U.S. Army Corps of Engineers built Lake Lanier to meet these needs. Laurel Ridge Trail explores the southern end of the lake, climbing through foothills of the Blue Ridge Mountains and exploring coves that are now claimed by the lake.

The trail begins as a cement walkway, passing behind the restrooms at the south end of Lower Overlook. A few steps after the brown-roofed stone restrooms, the path turns left and becomes a dirt treadway, descending into a small river valley with a deciduous forest. The path then begins a rock-strewn rise to the road. Crossing the road the path climbs some stone steps and zigzags through an entrance designed to allow only pedestrian traffic.

Directions

Take GA 400 North to Exit 14, Buford, Cumming. The exit passes under the overpass and then loops around. Turn right and travel 0.3 miles to GA 9. Turn right (by the Burger King and Wachovia) and travel 0.9 miles to Buford Dam Road. Turn right at the Shell station. In 4.8 miles the road makes a 90-degree left turn and crosses the dam. Laurel Ridge Trail crosses the road. Make your next left into Lower Overlook parking area, and park in the first parking area, near the restrooms.

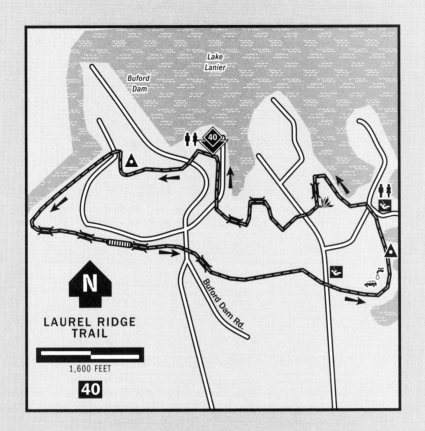

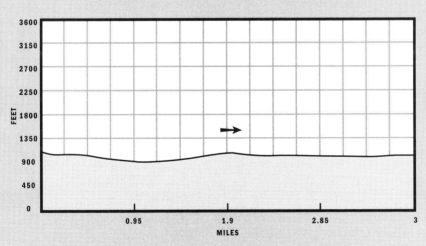

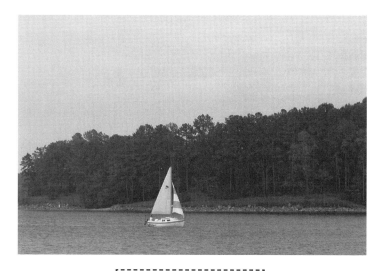

Sails unfurled on Lake Lanier

Relatively clear and wide, Laurel Ridge Trail winds through second-growth forest, mostly red maple and white oak accented by native dogwood in the clearings. As you approach the first park area, the trail makes a 90-degree turn to a wooden bridge. On the left is a playground. Turn right where the trail reaches a T-intersection as you approach a walled pavilion on your left, part of Upper Overlook Park. From the pavilion you'll have good views of the dam; there is also a monument created from a boring sample of rock drilled at the present-day site of the powerhouse. Return to the trail, which bears right at the end of the stone wall.

Descending at an easy grade, the trail makes another 90-degree right turn, descends more steeply, and for a short stretch is rocky, rooted, and deeply rutted. During the descent, observe how pines slowly become a larger part of the overall forest. A few benches have been added to allow tired hikers a rest. Just over 0.1 mile into the journey is a side trail down to a wooden overlook with benches that offers good winter views of Buford Dam. Returning to the path, turn right and descend the stairs. The trail then continues a steep descent along rooted and rocky terrain.

Ignore a trail to the left that leads down to an electric facility, but take a minute to climb the stairs to the overlook for a view of the Chattahoochee River basin and an excellent view of the entire Buford Dam. At 0.5 miles there is a road with parking that is closed while work is being done on the dam's generators. From here the trail is a steep, sometimes slippery hike to the Chattahoochee River basin. As the trail nears the bottom of the valley, it crosses a wooden bridge over a small stream. Look to your left to see the source of the stream, a spring in a boulder-strewn ridge. Less than 200 feet past the bridge, a side trail leads to Lower Pool. This portion of Buford Dam Park can be explored on the separate Lower Pool Trail (only a portion is covered in Bowmans Island).

Now following the east bank of the river birch–lined Chattahoochee, the well-defined trail is rocky, rooted, and poorly marked. After 0.25 miles the trail makes a 90-degree left turn, leaving the riverbank and climbing out of the valley. Ascending along the banks of a tributary, the trail repeatedly crosses the stream. Pine trees, weakened by pine beetles and brought down by wind, nearly block the trail at one point. The steady climb levels briefly where a wooden walkway crosses a wet area. Just before the end of the climb, a bridge with a bench allows hikers an up-close view of the stream cascading down a steep, moss-covered rock.

At just over 1.3 miles into the walk, the trail crosses Buford Dam Road again. Twin stone pillars mark the exit, and diagonally across the street two more stone pillars mark the entrance. After the pillars the trail bears left and reenters the forest. In the middle of a low ridge, the path parallels a stream on the left, eventually crossing a wooden bridge and climbing stairs to a level section that skirts a ridgetop.

Entering full sun in a field cleared for power lines at 1.6 miles, the trail descends and switchbacks down the hill to a flight of steps, where it again enters the cool, shaded forest. Immediately after entering the forest, you'll reach a small land bridge that crosses a gully, and a boardwalk that crosses a marsh. When you cross two paved roads that are currently closed to traffic, you are at the beginning of a series of parks with facilities and lake views. After passing a small playground to the right, the trail joins a sidewalk, zigzags past a pavilion, and descends steps. Turn right and look for a white rectangular blaze and a brown hiker sign as the path returns to compacted soil and eventually curves downhill to Lake Lanier. At the bottom of the hill, the path turns left, but continue straight to a dock (at 2.2 miles) that looks out over Lanier.

Almost six years after beginning the dam in 1950, the U.S. Army Corps of Engineers began filling Lake Lanier. It took almost three years to fill the 38,000-acre lake, whose stated primary purpose was to aid navigation downstream. Today the lake is managed for a variety of uses, including hydroelectric power, recreation, drinking water, and wildlife. The Corps of Engineers owns the entire shoreline, well above the "full pool" level of 1,070 feet, and manages most of this land in an effort to preserve both breeding grounds and habitat. Homeowners with boats must secure a special permit from the Corps to add a dock.

Return to the trail, turn right, then bear right down to a bridge across an arm of the lake. The trail begins a pattern, crossing a low ridge then dropping into a park near the lake. In the parks, watch for the white rectangular blaze or a brown hiker sign marking the trail. At 2.5 miles there are restrooms (closed in off-season) directly on the trail, with a spigot to refill water bottles. Just a few feet past this, a swinging bench invites hikers to spend a minute enjoying a lovely view of the lake. From here the trail follows the shoreline, crosses a low ridge, and comes into wetlands spanned by boardwalk-style bridges. A man-made pond attracts herons, kingfishers, foxes, and deer. There is an active beaver dam adjacent to the bridge over a marsh and creek in this area. Climbing to the top of the last ridge, the trail returns to the Lower Overlook parking area.

41 LITTLE MULBERRY TRAIL

 KEY AT-A-GLANCE INFORMATION

LENGTH: 6 miles

CONFIGURATION: Multiple loops

DIFFICULTY: Easy, except for the loop to the waterfalls and river valley, which are moderate

SCENERY: Waterfalls, unspoiled river valley, landscaped pond

EXPOSURE: Full sun, except on the hiking trail, which is shaded

TRAFFIC: Moderate

TRAIL SURFACE: Asphalt, except for the hiking trail, which is gravel

HIKING TIME: 3 hours

ACCESS: Open year-round, dawn–dusk

MAPS: At trailhead kiosk; USGS Hog Mountain and Auburn

FACILITIES: Restrooms, children's playground, small pond

SPECIAL COMMENTS: The observation deck at West Meadow is situated on one of the tallest hills in Gwinnett County.

UTM Trailhead Coordinates

UTM Zone (NAD27) 17S

Easting 0234346

Northing 3770007

IN BRIEF

This combined multiuse and pedestrian trail offers a 2-mile hike through an old-growth forest to unspoiled Table Rock Falls and then explores the adjacent river valley. Some long-distance scenic views make the multiuse section of the trail pleasing.

DESCRIPTION

Opened officially in September 2004, Little Mulberry Park is one part of a major park-building program the county began a few years ago. Among the new parks are McDaniel Farm (page 188), Tribble Mill (page 206), Yellow River, and Harbins Park.

From the trailhead kiosk, turn left toward a small pond, which the paved multiuse trail encircles. This is the smallest of the four distinct loops that make up the park's trails. A second phase will dramatically increase the number of trails available for hiking, mountain biking, and horseback riding. Pass a side trail to the parking lot; the trail begins to wind as it drops to the bed of the creek that forms the lake, crossing it on a wooden bridge. Just past the bridge is the spillway of the earthen dam. The trail begins an easy climb past a dock overlooking the lake. As the trail curves left, it passes picnic tables and a playground.

Directions ⟶

Take I-85 North to Exit 120, Hamilton Mill Road. Turn right on Hamilton Mill at the end of the ramp. At 0.1 mile, turn right on Brazalton Highway, travel 1.8 miles to Auburn Road (GA 124 East), and turn left on it at Walgreens. At 3.4 miles turn left on Fence Road and make another left 0.6 miles into Little Mulberry Park.

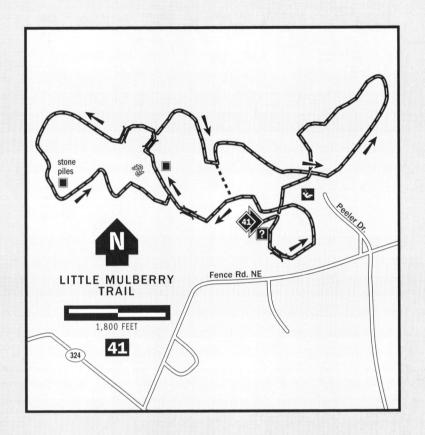

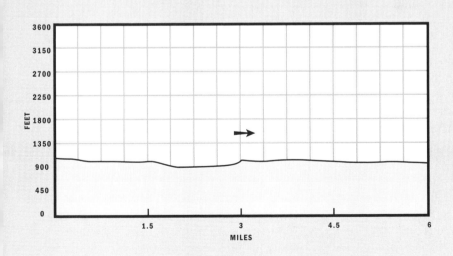

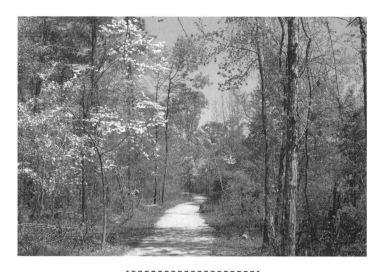

Dogwoods bloom in April.

Watch for a connecting trail on the right just past the playground. This rises to the second loop, surrounding West Meadow, a cleared area with an overlook at its center. Turn left and watch for a kiosk on your left at the end of a trail of pea-sized gravel that splits from the multiuse trail at 1.1 miles. On entering the full shade of the forest for the first time on the hike, the path switches to a wood chip–covered compacted-soil trail. Notice how the forest cools the air on even the hottest day. Just a few steps into the forest, the trail splits. We normally hike this section of the trail counterclockwise, so the return trail is on your left. Continue straight ahead, crossing a man-made rock-hop on a concrete culvert. The trail to the falls is on the left. After reading the interpretive sign, continue around to the left to Table Rock Falls at 1.3 miles. Dropping 30 feet to a flat rock, the stream spreads out along the rim, then freefalls another 15 feet, where it cascades, forming a small creek.

Return to the interpretive sign and continue straight, into a forest of American beech punctuated by an occasional red maple and shagbark hickory. Return to the main trail and turn left (it's more like a U-turn, really). After gaining a small hill, the trail begins the moderate-to-difficult descent into the river valley, quickly passing a stone bridge and Beech Tree Trail on the right. Descending the hill the trail switchbacks for an easy walk. Watch for a deep valley on the right as the trail descends then crosses a stone bridge over a gently babbling brook at 1.7 miles.

In the valley the trail levels off, running alongside a couple of streams before beginning to climb back to the hilltop. On the climb, watch for rock cairns in the forest. Built by Native Americans for an unknown reason (they hold neither bodies nor religious icons), many of these cairns are symmetrically stacked rocks, although some are scattered as if they had been vandalized. Protected within the park, there are hundreds of these mounds.

As you return to the top of the valley, bear left and continue to Beech Tree Trail, then turn right and exit the forest. The trail curves right as it climbs to the multiuse trail at 3.6 miles into the hike. Walk across West Meadow to the overlook (one of the highest points in Gwinnett County) for some excellent scenic views into the surrounding piedmont, then return to the multiuse trail and turn right. Walking downhill to a four-way intersection, head straight, then begin climbing to another high point. The trail curves around to the left, reaches a small hill, then begins an extended easy descent to the starting point. Go straight at the four-way intersection, then make a left on the connector trail. You'll see the trailhead kiosk on the right.

NEARBY ATTRACTIONS

Return to Auburn Road, turn left, and make a right on Dacula Highway. Watch for an impressive old home on the left. This is one of the earliest homes in the county, owned by Elisha Winn; it was the site of the first court held in Gwinnett County. Restored to its 1870s appearance, the home is usually open on Saturdays from 12:30 to 4:30 p.m.; phone (770) 822-5174.

42 MCDANIEL FARM PARK TRAIL

KEY AT-A-GLANCE INFORMATION

LENGTH: 2.3 miles

CONFIGURATION: Loop

DIFFICULTY: Easy

SCENERY: Meadowlands, Heritage Farm

EXPOSURE: Full sun

TRAFFIC: Moderate

TRAIL SURFACE: Paved with asphalt, except in the Heritage Farm

HIKING TIME: 1 hour; Heritage Farm tour adds 1 hour

ACCESS: Open year-round, dawn–dusk

MAPS: Available at trailhead and in interpreted farm area; USGS Norcross/Luxomni

FACILITIES: Restrooms at trailhead

SPECIAL COMMENTS: In spring the meadow is full of color.

IN BRIEF

McDaniel Farm Park is built around a subsistence farm similar to many of the farms in the area. In addition to the asphalt trail and a free self-guided tour of the farm, there is a heritage tour that is interpreted by docents on Tuesday, Thursday, and Saturday that takes in the farmhouse.

DESCRIPTION

When people think of antebellum Georgia, most picture the massive coastal cotton plantations. In the Atlanta area, however, most agriculture before the Civil War was subsistence farming, raising enough corn and wheat to meet only the family's needs. The grain products from these farms had to be cracked or ground before being consumed; wealthier planters coined the derogatory term "cracker" to describe the poorer farmers. Atlantans, though, were proud of the term: For more than 60 years, "Cracker" was the name of its minor league baseball team. Although the McDaniel family owned the farm from 1859 until it was given to the county after Archie McDaniel's death in 1999, the farm is set up as a 1930s farm might have been.

From the kiosk adjacent to the facilities, head left, following the asphalt path as it

UTM Trailhead Coordinates

UTM Zone (NAD27) 16S

Easting   0765349

Northing   3762218

Directions ⟶

Take I-85 North to Exit 103, Steve Reynolds Boulevard. Turn left at the end of the ramp and travel 1.1 miles, then turn right at Atlanta Toyota onto Old Norcross Road. At 0.6 miles turn left onto McDaniel Farm Road, just before the Land Rover dealership. Be careful—it's a divided highway that is not clearly marked. In 0.3 miles the road curves to the left and enters the parking lot for McDaniel Farm Park.

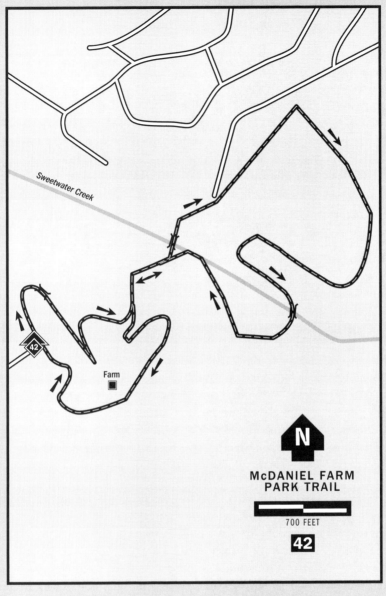

Sweetwater Creek

Farm

N

McDANIEL FARM
PARK TRAIL

700 FEET

42

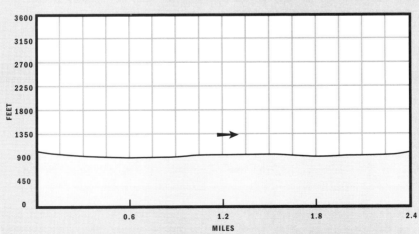

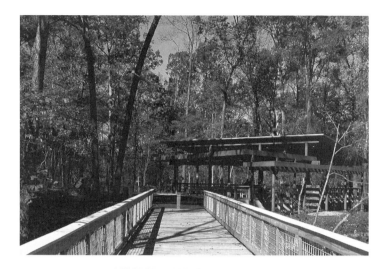

curves 180 degrees, passing a group shelter on the left before crossing a wooden bridge over a deep ravine. Watch for some larger trees here, including tulip poplar and oak. As you cross the bridge, the farm's entrance is directly ahead. Guided tours are given every Tuesday, Thursday, and Saturday at 10 a.m. and 2 p.m. and cost $3. If you can't make the tour, pick up a brochure from the metal pail hanging just inside the barn on the left wall. We strongly recommend the walking tour because it gives visitors access to the farmhouse, which is the most interesting building on the farm.

The lower level of the barn is used to house animals—cows, horses, mules, and pigs. The upper floor, or loft, was used to store feed, which could be dropped down to the animals through specially built chutes. On either side are two additional covered areas where a farmer could store machinery or extra feed he couldn't get in the loft. Also notice that the barn has a lot of open spaces in the building; these allowed the air that accumulated in the mild Georgia winters to circulate through the barn all year.

Continue to the farmhouse straight ahead. There is a chicken coop (henhouse) to the right and a smokehouse to the left. The hens would have been kept for their eggs and not raised for consumption. Smoked or salted meat cured in the smokehouse could be stored for months without refrigeration. After the Civil War, the McDaniels built the farmhouse, which is directly in front of you; it reflects the fact that the family enjoyed prosperity. For the McDaniels, cotton became a cash crop after the Civil War, adding to the farm's income.

Notice an old pear tree and pecan tree close to the house and a Chinese chestnut a bit farther back. In front and on the far side are post and white oak. The lawn is swept—there is no grass—because it would take time to tend the

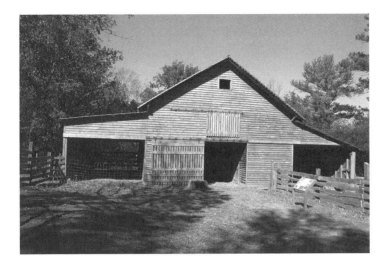

Reconstructed barn

lawn. Inside the home, photos of each family member adorn the rooms in which they slept, and letters written home by the boys during World War II are simply addressed "McDaniel, Duluth, Georgia."

Circle the farmhouse and return to the barn. Once through the barn, turn right on the asphalt path. Known as Cross Park Trail, the path begins a moderate descent to Sweetwater Creek, passing a trail to the parking lot on the right at 0.4 miles. At the bottom of the hill, just before the bridge over the creek, the return trail from the loop enters from the right.

This portion of the path was once a county roadway, but almost all evidence of this fact has been obliterated. Only in the vicinity of the farmhouse is the road evident. From the bridge the path begins to climb, bearing left at 0.7 miles at a three-way intersection. The path continues to a maintenance area, where it turns right to become Wildflower Trail. From a ridge just under a mile into the hike, you can see commercial development off to the left. At this point the trail begins an easy descent as it curves left toward a forested area with a variety of large pines.

After the trees, meadowland, where the McDaniels once planted cotton fields, has been planted to provide color in the spring. Cotton was grown on the farm only until the 1920s, when the boll weevil infestation reached Gwinnett County. After about 1925 the McDaniels planted corn, okra, and butter beans in these fields.

When a path heads off to the right at 1.4 miles, continue straight to another pedestrian bridge over Sweetwater Creek, less than 0.1 mile ahead. After the bridge the trail wraps around to the right and returns to Cross Park Trail. Turn left and climb the hill to an alternate return trail to the parking lot at 2 miles. Turn left on the level path as it swings around McDaniel Farm's outer perimeter.

The small house on the right at 2.2 miles was used by the tenant farmer who worked on McDaniel Farm in exchange for food and a small amount of money ($5 for all the work he did for a winter in the 1930s, according to a display inside the house). Notice the outhouse adjacent to the tenant's house. Continue on the trail to the parking lot.

NEARBY ATTRACTIONS

Turn left onto old Norcross Road, then turn left at the first traffic light. Gwinnett Place Mall is on your right. Gwinnett Place features major anchor stores like Sears and Macy's and many smaller upscale shops. For rail fans, return to Pleasant Hill Road and turn right, then turn right at Buford Highway for the Southeastern Railway Museum.

STONE MOUNTAIN LOOP 43

IN BRIEF

This loop trail takes visitors to most of the major attractions at Stone Mountain.

DESCRIPTION

After parking, return to the sidewalk in front of Confederate Hall and turn left, walking Stone Mountain Loop counterclockwise. Follow the sidewalk 0.2 miles to a trestle for Stone Mountain Railroad. Walk under the trestle and turn left, entering the forest for the first time. At just under 0.4 miles, there is a path to the right, almost hidden in the summer months. Descend a few steps to two polished granite "bridges" across a creek. Return to the main trail and turn left.

Continue on the orange connector trail until a marked right-hand turn at 0.6 miles. This is the entrance to the nature center, which has an interpreted display of plants native to Georgia. Among the trees are mulberry and white oak. Plants include strawberry, Christmas fern, trumpet creeper, fragrant sumac, and beautyberries. As you walk through the garden keep a small building on your left and continue to the other side. Mulberry trees and a railed bridge at 0.7 miles indicate the end of the nature center.

KEY AT-A-GLANCE INFORMATION

LENGTH: 5.5 miles
CONFIGURATION: Loop
DIFFICULTY: Easy
SCENERY: Multiple views of Stone Mountain and the Confederate Memorial, the world's largest carving, a gristmill, covered bridge, streams, and lakeshore
EXPOSURE: Full sun in the area of the memorial and in multiple areas where the trail runs on granite, mostly shaded elsewhere
TRAFFIC: Heavy between Confederate Hall and Sky Lift, light elsewhere
TRAIL SURFACE: Compacted soil, Chattahoochee stone, granite
HIKING TIME: 2.5 hours
ACCESS: Open year-round
MAPS: Request the hiking map when purchasing your parking pass ($7); an additional map is available at Confederate Hall; USGS Stone Mountain
FACILITIES: Restrooms at the trailhead and at most attractions; playgrounds, picnic tables
SPECIAL COMMENTS: Scouts can earn merit badges for hiking this trail. Stop by Confederate Hall for details. While inside the park, be sure to visit the Antebellum Plantation and the Carillon Bells, the only major attractions not on the Stone Mountain Loop. Phone (770) 498-5690.

Directions

Take I-285 East to Exit 39B, Stone Mountain Freeway East (Snellville, Athens) and drive 7.8 miles to the exit for Stone Mountain East Gate. The road curves right, then comes to a gate. After the gate, this road is known as Jefferson Davis Drive. Continue 1 mile to where the road splits. Bear left and merge onto Robert E. Lee Boulevard. Follow it 1 mile to Confederate Hall. Turn left and park.

UTM Trailhead Coordinates

UTM Zone (NAD27) 16S

Easting   0762706

Northing   3744591

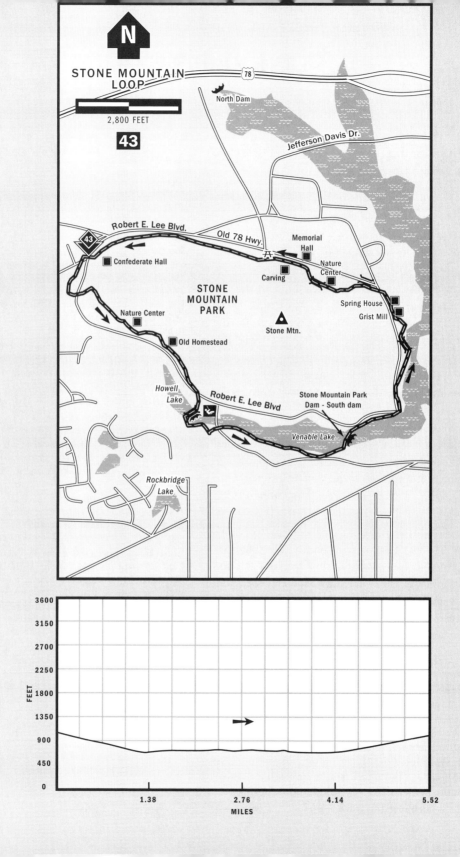

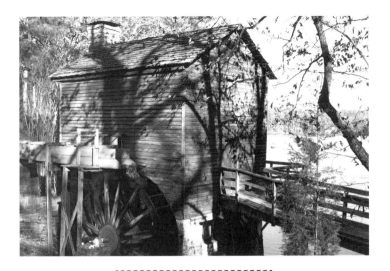

Grist Mill in Stone Mountain Park

After crossing a stream, the footpath bears right, coming to an intersection with Cherokee (Red) Trail. Turn right and continue to the remains of a house at 1 mile. You can see the roofline cut in the chimney about two-thirds of the way to the top. There are wire cuts in a tree on the opposite site of the house as well. The path bears right at 1.3 miles, climbs a set of railroad-tie steps, and crosses Robert E. Lee Boulevard. Keep a green-fenced playground on your right as you reenter the forest. The trail circles the playground, turning left on a gravel road, then crossing the dam that forms Howell Lake. Step down into the cement overflow, then climb up a similar step on the other side. As the path bears left, there is a railed bridge crossing over a strong creek at 1.5 miles. Just 0.1 mile later, the path crosses Stonewall Jackson Drive.

Venable Lake, on your left, is named for Sam Venable, who ran the quarry early in the 20th century. About halfway around the lake, the trail bears right, crosses a beautiful stream with cascades flowing over a series of large rocks, and then bears left to return to the lakeshore. At 2.5 miles the footpath makes a hard right turn, crossing an earthen dam and turning right on the far side of the lake. On your right is the largest body of water in the park, Stone Mountain Lake.

Just before 2.8 miles, Stone Mountain Loop rises around a rock outcropping, turns inland, makes a right just before the road, and falls to a creek. The trail becomes undefined crossing granite outcroppings, but watch for white blazes on the rock. The number of trails to the lakeshore increase, and the covered bridge comes into view at 3.2 miles. W. W. King built the lattice bridge in 1891. Originally, the bridge spanned the Oconee River in Athens, but when the Georgia Department of Transportation replaced the bridge in 1965, they offered it to Stone Mountain Park for $1. The park accepted and moved the bridge to its present site at a cost of $18,000.

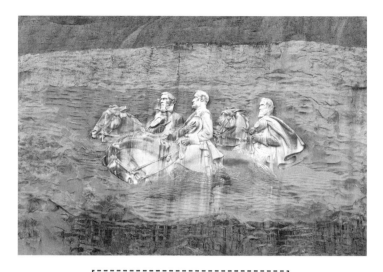

Confederate Memorial at Stone Mountain

The footpath falls to the lakeshore and crosses an outflow on two granite tablets. The path runs adjacent to the lake, inches above the water level and with a granite wall on the left. Watch for two sets of two granite hearts put in the pathway by an energetic stonemason. As the path curves to the left, moving away from the lake, concrete walkways replace the trail at 3.6 miles. The network of walkways offers views of the Stone Mountain gristmill, but head for the mill-wheel and a boardwalk that runs next to the mill for a close-up look at the structure. At the far end of the boardwalk, turn right and continue uphill to a granite sluice and springhouse. Keeping the sluice on your right, cross a field and small steam, turn left, and climb to Robert E. Lee Boulevard.

After you cross the road, the trail winds its way through second-growth forest, mostly oak and beech, then climbs railroad-tie steps to cross the tracks at 4 miles. A nature garden established by the Atlanta branch of the National League of American Pen Women in 1961 is on the left. After you pass under the alpine-style Skylift cables, keep a small garage at 4.4 miles on your right as you circle to the right and climb to Memorial Plaza. As the path curves to the left, it turns to Chattahoochee stone, and the carving comes into view for the first time.

The massive relief sculpture of Jefferson Davis, Robert E. Lee, and Stonewall Jackson is carved in the world's largest piece of solid rock and represents the work of three sculptors over a period of 56 years. Gutzon Borglum began working on a concept for the sculpture in 1916, although actual carving did not begin until 1923. He quickly ran into problems, first with his system to project the carving onto the mountain, then with just about everybody involved in the project. He left Georgia just ahead of a police car. Next came Augustus Lukeman, who gave up on Borglum's original concept and blasted it off the face of the mountain. Lukeman had made significant progress on the current carving when the project failed to meet its deadline in 1928. The partially completed carving sat for 30 years at the intersection of two rural highways.

When the State of Georgia purchased the land in 1958, they immediately set out to complete the work, hiring sculptor Walker Hancock, although Roy Faulkner, a former marine with no experience carving stone before working for Mr. Hancock, did most of the work. Dedicated in 1970, the project was declared complete in 1972. On the right, across an open field, is Memorial Hall, which contains an excellent museum that highlights the mountain, the sculptors, and some local history.

Stone Mountain Loop turns left, crosses railroad tracks, and bears right, reentering the forest. At 4.5 miles the railroad depot is on the right, on the far side of some picnic tables and the tracks. It is a re-creation of the Atlanta depot that Sherman destroyed in his 1864 March to the Sea. General admission tickets allow access to all attractions. Because of seasonal and hourly variations, check **www.stonemountainpark.com** for current pricing information. Behind the depot is the recently added Crossroads, an area of shops designed to resemble a frontier village, with areas called the Treehouses and the Great Barn, and a 4-D theater with a film about the Southern art of storytelling

Past the picnic tables, the trail runs between the mountain and the railroad and continues in a shortleaf and loblolly pine forest on a frequently rocky trail, occasionally moving into full sun when it climbs on solid granite outcroppings of the mountain. The red-blazed Cherokee Trail heads off to the right at the marked intersection at 5.2 miles, then Stone Mountain Loop runs adjacent to the tracks as it crosses a paved road and enters the Confederate Hall complex.

44 STONE MOUNTAIN MOUNTAINTOP TRAIL

KEY AT-A-GLANCE INFORMATION

LENGTH: 2.4 miles

CONFIGURATION: Out-and-back, with a small loop at the top of the mountain

DIFFICULTY: Difficult; extended periods of boulder climbing on the path, nearby vertical drops near the path, and extremely slippery conditions for days after a rain

SCENERY: 360-degree vista of the Georgia piedmont, including long-distance views of Atlanta, Buckhead, and Decatur

EXPOSURE: Full sun for the entire hike

TRAFFIC: Heavy

TRAIL SURFACE: Granite rock and boulders

HIKING TIME: 2 hours, including a small museum at the top

ACCESS: Open year-round, dawn–dusk; fee required

MAPS: Available at both entrances and at Confederate Hall; USGS Stone Mountain

FACILITIES: Restrooms, candy and soda machines

SPECIAL COMMENTS: Stone Mountain Mountaintop Trail is one of the most scenic and historic trails in the Southeastern United States.

UTM Trailhead Coordinates

UTM Zone (NAD27) 16S

Easting 0762706

Northing 3744591

IN BRIEF

This trail climbs on solid granite and through boulder fields to the top of Stone Mountain, some 780 feet above the surrounding Georgia piedmont.

DESCRIPTION

Climb Mountaintop Trail to the top of Stone Mountain and you are walking through 200 years of American history, 400 years of European history, thousands of years of Native American history, and millions of years in geological history.

Formed 7 miles beneath the Earth's surface more than 350 million years ago, Stone Mountain is what geologists call a pluton. Molten lava, created by the massive collision of tectonic plates during the formation of the Blue Ridge Mountains, forced its way into an underlying fold over many millions of years. The east side of the mountain was the first side to be formed. Stone Mountain granite is significantly different than the underlying Lithonia granite belt that runs east and south of the mountain. Archaic American Indian sites dating back 8,000 years have been found near the mountain, in addition to woodland American Indian sites, Moundbuilder sites, and Creek villages.

Directions

Take I-285 East to Exit 39B, Stone Mountain Freeway East (Snellville, Athens) and travel 7.8 miles to the exit for Stone Mountain East Gate. The road curves right, then comes to a gate, where you pay an $8 parking fee. Past here, this road is known as Jefferson Davis Drive. Continue 1 mile before the road splits. Bear right and merge onto Robert E. Lee Boulevard. Follow it 1 mile to Confederate Hall. Turn left and park.

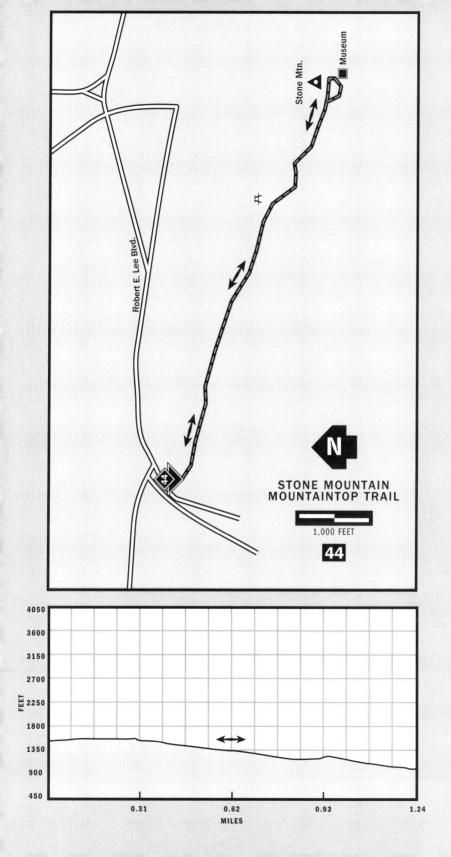

STONE MOUNTAIN
MOUNTAINTOP TRAIL

1,000 FEET

44

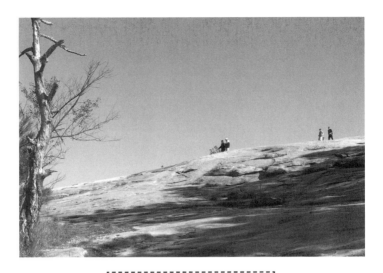

When Spanish explorers first visited the mountain (in about 1560), they called the monadnock Crystal Mountain because of the quartz found around the base and embedded in the mountain. The Creek climbed the trail to the mountaintop, frequently using the site to meet with nearby Cherokees. In 1790 Colonel Marinus Willet met Creek chiefs at the top of the mountain and escorted them to New York to meet with President George Washington.

Settlers moving west along Hightower Trail called the peak Rock Fort Mountain because earlier Woodland Indians had built a wall around the top. Over time the name was shortened to Rock Mountain. Baptist minister Adiel Sherwood, one of the founders of Mercer College (Macon), renamed the peak Stone Mountain. Large-scale granite quarrying began about 1847, the same year the nearby town changed its name from New Gibraltar to Stone Mountain. Civil War battles briefly raged near the mountain in July 1864, and the Left Wing of Sherman's army passed just to the north of the mountain in November 1864 on the March to the Sea. In 1958 the state purchased the mountain and surrounding land and turned it into a state park. One of the first buildings in the park was Confederate Hall, which is on your left on the approach to the railroad crossing that marks the start of the trail.

Once across the tracks, the trail begins its climb, easy at first but quickly increasing in grade. There are no level or downhill sections until the return trip. At 0.3 miles into the hike, power lines come in from the left and follow near the rock path to the top of the mountain. During this part of the ascent, there are boulders spread across the path; climbing them can take a while.

Just over 0.6 miles into the hike is a picnic shelter. Look closely on the right to see a historic barbecue grill. From this point on is the steepest portion of the climb. Keep your eyes on the trail: embedded in the granite a short distance past the shelter is an engraved plaque that marks Cherokee Trail, a historic pathway that crosses Mountaintop Trail at this point. Just a few steps up from the plaque, parallel metal railings help unsteady visitors up a particularly steep portion of the footpath, but good hikers can easily bypass these structures by bearing left at a split in the trail before the railings. Follow this trail through a large boulder field, watching for Bubble Gum Rock, where visitors have left their chewing gum for many years.

Now the trail has climbed far enough up to allow stunning views of the relatively level piedmont surrounding Stone Mountain. Moving to the left, closer to the sheer northern face where the carving is, the trail passes a series of metal structures attached to the mountain. These were some of the infrastructure added to the mountain to support the men carving the sculpture. Rising toward the peak, the trail passes near a vernal ("spring") pool with red moss. These pools fill with rainwater in the spring and literally come to life. Tiny fairy shrimp, whose lifespan is measured in days, not years, are born, reproduce, and die. When the pools dry up during the winter or in heavy drought years, animals and wind spread the eggs to other vernal pools.

As we reached the mountaintop, tour guide Matt Wood met us to show us some of the highlights. Walking near the steep north face of the mountain, where we had an incredible long-distance view, we listened as Matt told us of Elias Nour, who was frequently called to rescue people from the cliff face. His legendary exploits, some of which are discussed in David B. Freeman's book about Stone Mountain, *Carved in Stone*, include pushing a burning car off the face of the mountain as a stunt to attract people to the partially completed mountain.

At the top of the mountain is a dual-purpose structure: it is both the dock for the Skylift, and a small museum with some good information on the natural history of the mountain. As we walked toward the structure we passed the highest point of the mountain. Yellow paint on the northeast side of some rock was the next point of interest. In the early 1920s, before airplanes had directional systems, the rock was painted with the word "Atlanta" and a huge arrow pointing toward the city. Stone Mountain, which was visible for 50 miles on a clear day, was the guiding point for fliers from the northeast. At the museum/Skylift, Matt told us that the alpine-style lift was one of the park's first attractions. As we began to circle back to our starting point, we saw a white line designating a drivable road down the mountain. A large, fenced-off area protects the fragile habitat of the fairy shrimp and other species. At the end of the loop, turn left and retrace your steps to the car.

NEARBY ATTRACTIONS

Confederate Hall, phone (770) 498-5658), which is the building at the base of the mountain, has extensive information on the geology and environment of Stone Mountain, plus an excellent display on the (Civil) War in Georgia narrated by Hal Holbrook. Stone Mountain village offers a large number of eclectic shops with various merchandise.

45 SUWANEE GREENWAY

IN BRIEF

This hike follows the floodplain of Suwanee Creek from George F. Pierce Park to Suwanee Creek Park.

DESCRIPTION

It is no understatement to call Suwanee Greenway the environmental success story of the Atlanta area. Destroyed by source-point pollution, Suwanee Creek was known locally as Black Creek. Bona Allen Tannery, located on the creek in Buford, Georgia, was founded in 1873 and pumped untreated chemicals used in the tanning process into the river. Acid, lime, and dyes all made their way into Suwanee Creek, killing virtually all living creatures and creating a 15-mile environmental disaster area. When the tannery closed in the 1970s, it was estimated that the river could take 100 years to return to a normal state. Today the river has risen from the dead, some 30 years after the factory closed.

Stretching from George F. Pierce Park (a 300-acre Gwinnett County Park) to the new Suwanee Creek Park (an 85-acre park developed by the city of Suwanee), the Greenway offers visitors the chance to hike, bike, walk, run, or skate along a 4-mile, level, paved trail; additional paved and gravel hiking is available

UTM Trailhead Coordinates

UTM Zone (NAD27) 16S

Easting 0768875

Northing 3769537

Directions ➤

Take I-85 North to Exit 111, GA 317/ Lawrenceville-Suwanee Road. Turn left on GA 317 and travel 2.1 miles to Buford Highway (US 23). Turn right and go 0.3 miles to the first traffic light, then turn right into George F. Pierce Park. Travel 1 mile to the parking area and make a left down the first aisle. Park at the far end of this aisle, near an embankment.

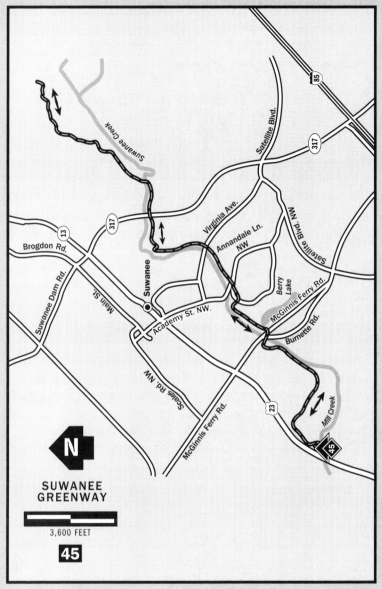

SUWANEE
GREENWAY

3,600 FEET

45

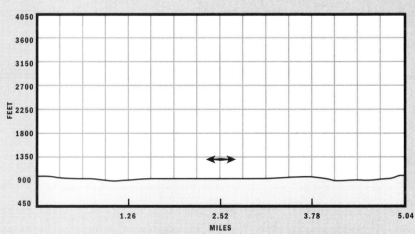

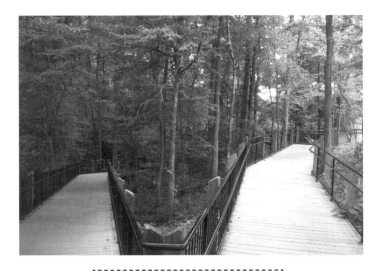

Unusual ramp to McGinness Ferry Road

in the parks at either end. Between the two parks, Suwanee Creek has a wide range of native and nonnative trees and shrubs, waterfowl, and wildlife.

Our hike begins at the south end of Pierce Park. Although we love the Greenway, by beginning here it gives us at least a little time away from the cyclists and in-line skaters who dominate the paved portion of the hike. Climbing up the embankment, turn left after entering the mostly oak forest. We ran into a rooster not very far along the trail. The unblazed but easily followed footpath descends into the watershed of a tributary of Suwanee Creek, winding as it climbs to a paved road at 0.3 miles. Turn right and follow the road 200 feet to the nature trail sign, then turn left. A short way down this compacted-soil trail is a Rules of the Road sign that indicates the start of the multiuse trail.

The forest is replaced by manicured grass as you enter full sun, but forest returns at 0.5 miles. The trail becomes a gravel road and continues an easy descent. On the left a wetland stretches across a low floodplain between the road embankment and Suwanee Creek. Waterfowl and larger predators inhabit this floodplain throughout the year. Just past a bench on the right, the road makes a sharp right turn and continues skirting the creek until it makes another right turn onto a long bridge with wooden slats and a metal railing. For the first time, the trail enters the wetland, with some excellent long-distance views. At 1.2 miles the trail turns left on a wooden bridge and crosses Suwanee Creek, again with some great river views. About midway across the bridge it turns right, then comes to an asphalt path. Bear left and continue across another wooden bridge. At the end of the bridge, the trail bears left, quickly coming to an underpass at 1.5 miles, where the trail narrows.

Emerging from the underpass, Suwanee Greenway turns left and begins to meander through the manicured grass of the wide floodplain of Suwanee Creek to head west, following the river as it curves to the left and begins to flow south-ward. At 2.2 miles the pathway crosses Martin's Farm Road, and a side trail on the left takes you to a parking area with some playground equipment. The Green-way changes noticeably, with wetlands frequently engulfing the path that has almost imperceptibly turned west again. This habitat, which also serves as a breeding grounds and a rest stop for migratory birds, provides dramatic proof of the recovery of both the creek and the nearby wetlands. Among the species that make use of the once-polluted creek and wetlands are great blue herons, black vultures, red-tailed and red-shouldered hawks, osprey, and the American bald eagle. Watch for typical water-loving grasses, such as goldenrod and cattails, and trees, such as the river birch and white ash.

The Greenway then enters a swamp created by an active beaver dam. As the paved road rises, Annandale Lane dead-ends into Suwanee Greenway at 2.7 miles. Following the road the trail runs above an area of immense trees. In addition to varieties of oak, there are loblolly and shortleaf pine, tulip poplar, sweetgum, and red maple. A ramped, switchbacking wooden walkway takes you up to McGinniss Ferry Road. At the road the trail turns right, using the curbed sidewalk on the bridge to cross Suwanee Creek, then it turns right again, easily curving right and descending to the creek, passing under the bridge. As the path comes out the other side, it curves to the right again and rises to Burnette Road parking lot, where it makes a 90-degree left turn.

From McGinnis Ferry to Suwanee Creek Park, the paved trail repeatedly rises on low wooden bridges to cross thriving, sensitive wetland areas. Once again, be ready to see a good deal of wildlife, although we spotted only smaller mammals, including raccoons and rabbits. At 4 miles the last bridge ends and the trail splits in a garden of native plantings. The trail on the right is a quick, refreshing thigh-stretch to Suwanee Creek Park, while the trail straight ahead is more gradual, intended for cyclists.

The city of Suwanee has created a wonderful environment in the park. The paved trail explores a small knoll that is vastly different than the Greenway. At a four-way intersection with a parking lot immediately on the right, go straight to explore the park. Pavilions and picnic tables dot the landscape as the trail crosses the entrance road at 4.3 miles. As the pathway approaches Buford Highway, it makes a U-turn deep in a forested cove on a wooden bridge across a gully, then rises and parallels the roadway to a parking lot. Walk past the pavilion on the far end of the parking lot and turn right.

An overlook allows folks to view Suwanee Creek from above, then the footpath continues on, curving to the right to an unobstructed (although decidedly suburban) view at 4.7 miles. The trail loops to the right, returning to the inbound trail. Turn left and retrace your steps to the car.

46 TRIBBLE MILL TRAIL

KEY AT-A-GLANCE INFORMATION

LENGTH: 3 miles

CONFIGURATION: Loop

DIFFICULTY: Easy

SCENERY: 2 lakes, forested wetlands

EXPOSURE: Full sun

TRAFFIC: Moderate

TRAIL SURFACE: Paved asphalt

HIKING TIME: 1.5 hours

ACCESS: Open year-round, dawn–dusk

MAPS: At both entrances; USGS Lawrenceville

FACILITIES: Restrooms, picnic tables with grills and pavilions, playground, meadow area with wildflowers, amphitheater

SPECIAL COMMENTS: A recent addition to the Gwinnett County park system, Tribble Mill is still only partially complete. Within the park there is an additional 18 miles of mountain bike trails.

UTM Trailhead Coordinates

UTM Zone (NAD27) 17S

Easting 0230748

Northing 3756012

IN BRIEF

This multiuse trail explores one of the two man-made lakes and a portion of the 800-acre Tribble Mill Park.

DESCRIPTION

The Grayson area is in the first part of Gwinnett that was settled by farmers from the east. It was originally incorporated into the State of Georgia in 1784 as part of Franklin County, but ceded when Gwinnett County was formed in 1818. Grayson was founded in 1881 under the name Berkeley, which they changed to Grayson in 1902 to avoid having two Georgia towns with the same name.

Two man-made lakes—Ozora Lake (109 acres) and Chandler Lake (40 acres)—form the centerpiece of Tribble Mill Park, and the paved, multiuse trail circles most of Ozora Lake. From the parking lot you have a good long-distance view up the lake. At the road, turn right on the trail, which begins to rise as it parallels Tribble Mill Parkway. It dips into a forest of pine and dogwood, quickly returning to the parkway. The second time the trail descends, it begins to drop steeply past a post designed to prevent vehicular traffic from entering the multiuse trail.

Directions

Take I-285 East to Exit 39B, Stone Mountain Freeway East (Snellville, Athens), and drive 16.3 miles to GA 84 (begin watching for it after crossing Scenic Highway [GA 124] in downtown Snellville). Turn left and travel 5.6 miles to a four-way stop at New Hope Road. Turn right and travel 0.5 miles, making a right on Tribble Mill Parkway. After entering the park, turn left in the first parking lot and return to the trail.

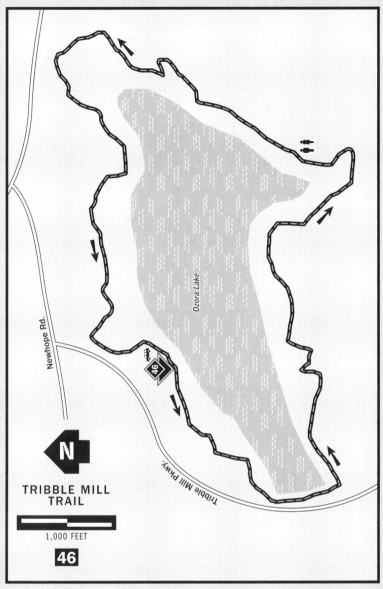

**TRIBBLE MILL
TRAIL**

1,000 FEET

46

Newhope Rd.

Tribble Mill Pkwy.

Ozora Lake

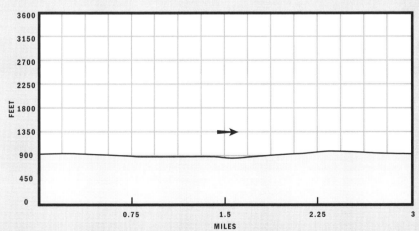

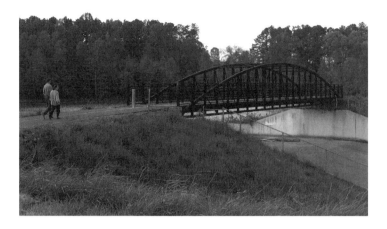

Overflow dam for Lake Ozora

The trail parallels the lakeshore, running above it to offer some good long-distance views, and the forest diversifies. By the time the trail makes a hard left at 0.4 miles, white and post oak, American beech, maple, and elm have all joined the loblolly–shortleaf pine forest. An overlook made from granite, with steel seats, has a somewhat blocked view of the lake and Ozora Meadow in the distance. Turn left at 0.8 miles, where the trail splits, and there is a much better overlook on the right. When the trails rejoin, turn left; the pathway continues to bear left, following the curve of the lake. As the lakeshore begins to curve back around to the right, the trail makes a corresponding curve, crossing an earthen dam with a spillway at 1.3 miles.

After the dam, take the trail to the right as it continues to follow the lakeshore. On your left, past the amphitheater, is Ozora Meadow, an open field where kids can play. After the field and the children's playground, turn left and climb to the restrooms. To return to the main trail, make the next right, then another right at the parking lot. When you reach the lakeshore turn left, entering full shade for the first time on the hike. The trail curves left and follows a stream on the right to a boardwalk bridge. Trails, which allow you to explore the area below the boardwalk, can be accessed before the boardwalk or from a sitting area on the left after the bridge.

Following the bridge the trail begins a good thigh-burning climb to the top of a small ridge. Multiple mountain-bike paths cross the trail here, and you can take any of these to further explore the area. The trail begins to curve more, falling to a roadbed at 2.1 miles and then continuing an easy climb. Just 0.2 miles later the trail crosses a second road, curves right, then makes a U-turn as it begins to descend. After crossing a wooden bridge with metal railings, the path turns right as it runs adjacent to Tribble Mill Parkway under the Julian W. Archer Sr. Bridge and returns to the parking lot.

NEARBY ATTRACTIONS

Once you're done hiking Tribble Mill, follow the same route back, but turn left at Scenic Highway (GA 124). At Anniston Road, turn right then left on Juhan Road. A paved 1-mile multiuse trail (a good place to let the kids pedal off some steam) can be accessed from the first parking lot on the left. If you want to try the 5.7-mile mountain bike trail, which can be hiked, or the equestrian trail, use the second parking lot, also on the left.

On the north end of the multiuse trail is a meadow and "council area" that is planted with native grasses and wildflowers, and an observation deck that has good views of the Yellow River. On the day we visited, children were playing in the river near the observation deck. Continuing past the end of the pavement, a pedestrian trail climbs a hill with a creek on the left, loops back to the equestrian trail, and drops with the same creek on the right, returning to the paved multiuse trail.

The bike paths form a double-loop, one south and one north of the mountain-biking parking area. The southern loop has less elevation change and is slightly shorter. The northern loop climbs out of the river valley to nearby knolls.

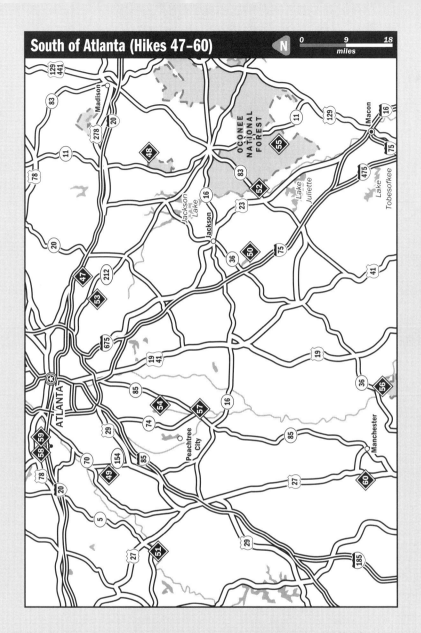

SOUTH OF ATLANTA

47 ARABIA MOUNTAIN TRAIL

KEY AT-A-GLANCE INFORMATION

LENGTH: 5.1 miles

CONFIGURATION: Double loop with connecting trail

DIFFICULTY: Moderate

SCENERY: Long-distance mountain-top views, 2 lakes, forested wetlands, and small streams

EXPOSURE: Full sun with some areas of partial shade, including the area around Arabia Lake

TRAFFIC: Moderate

TRAIL SURFACE: Stone, compacted dirt, some pavement

HIKING TIME: 3 hours

ACCESS: Open year-round, dawn–dusk

MAPS: Available at nature center and both trailhead kiosks; USGS Redan, Conyers

FACILITIES: Restrooms; nature center; picnic tables, including 2 on the hike near Arabia Lake

SPECIAL COMMENTS: Arabia Mountain Trail is connected to Stonecrest Mall in Lithonia via a paved multiuse trail; this hike follows a small part of this. Formed by metamorphosed granite, the mountains are much older than nearby Stone Mountain.

UTM Trailhead Coordinates

UTM Zone (NAD27) 16S

Easting   0766671

Northing   3727919

IN BRIEF

This hike explores the Arabia Mountain area, composed of three distinct "mountains" made of Lithonia gneiss. From the top of Bradley Mountain, the trail is not marked, but it is easy to pick up near the bottom.

DESCRIPTION

On first sight, Arabia Mountain will look a lot like Stone Mountain because both are rock outcrops. There is a difference, however, in the type and age of the stone, and in the size of the two formations. Arabia Mountain is made of Lithonia gneiss, metamorphosed granite that is 700 million years old, whereas Stone Mountain is made of granite half that age. Aside from that, the barren landscape is surprisingly similar. Both formations have vernal pools and Georgia oaks, and they supported quarrying operations from the mid-1800s on. Like Stone Mountain, Arabia Mountain is near a crossroads. In fact, the nearby city of Lithonia ("stone place" in Latin) was originally called Crossroads.

From the parking lot, walk toward the elongated wooden trailhead kiosk and a split-rail fence. After traversing a stunted-pine forest,

Directions

Take I-20 West to Evans Mill Road. At the end of the ramp, turn right on Evans Mill Road. At 0.1 mile continue straight through a traffic light on Woodrow Drive (Evans Mill turns right). Continue on Woodrow Drive 0.9 miles to Klondike Road. Turn right and watch for the Davidson-Arabia Mountain Nature Center on the right at 1.2 miles, but continue on to the Arabia Mountain parking area on the left at 2.1 miles. If this lot is full, use the nature center parking as overflow.

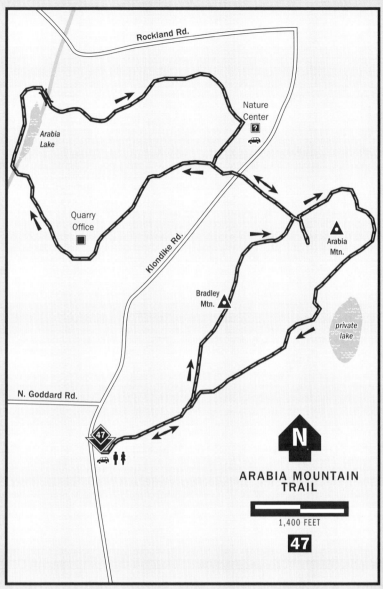

Rockland Rd.

Nature
Center

Arabia
Lake

Quarry
Office

Klondike Rd.

Arabia
Mtn.

Bradley
Mtn.

private
lake

N. Goddard Rd.

47

N

**ARABIA MOUNTAIN
TRAIL**

1,400 FEET

47

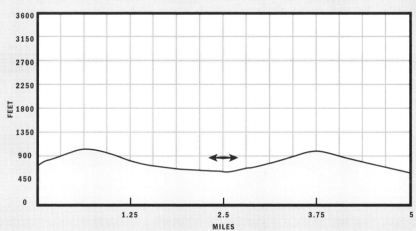

3600					
3150					
2700					
2250					
FEET
1800					
1350					
900					
450					
0					

1.25   2.5   3.75   5

MILES

the path curves left, dipping through a low area with more pine trees, then begins the easy climb to the top of the first hill, Bradley Mountain. Knee-high cairns guide hikers to the top of the mountain, and not very far into the hike visitors are rewarded with an astounding view of the rolling hills of the Georgia piedmont. Atop Bradley Mountain, 0.6 miles into the hike, you have a 360-degree view, with Arabia Mountain ahead on the right.

Facing Arabia Mountain at the top of Bradley Mountain, look down to your left at about 10 o'clock. An unmarked stone path with trees on either side will lead you down to an opening in the trees with a glass-covered box explaining the flora of Arabia Mountain. If you can't find the correct path, don't worry. Simply walk to the tree line at the bottom of the mountain and follow it until you come to the opening. When you pass through the opening, turn left at 1 mile on an old roadbed and walk to Klondike Road. After crossing the road, turn left on the asphalt-paved multiuse trail, which connects Arabia Mountain to Stonecrest Mall in Lithonia. Follow the paved trail across a bridge and turn right on a wide, sandy road covered with pine leaves that leads to a three-way intersection at 1.2 miles. Turn left and continue on this path until it turns into solid rock; you will immediately see the first cairn.

As the trail meanders over the rock, watch for areas that have been quarried and for indigenous plant life, such as red moss. At 1.4 miles, a large indentation that is normally wet has an interpretive sign about the frogs living there. From here the trail turns left, then makes a right and comes to a one-story building of Lithonia gneiss. This is the remains of the old quarry office and weigh station, just over 1.7 miles into the hike. The paved-asphalt trail is directly in front of you, but turn right, keeping the stone building on your left, and take the wide, partially shaded pine leaf–covered road that turns into South Lake Trail. As the trail returns to full sun, the cairns guide you to the top of an unnamed stone knoll. From your vantage point here, look for more cairns, a picnic table, and a pavilion to the left as you face north. This is where the trail enters a mostly to fully shaded pine forest adjacent to Arabia Lake.

Quickly reaching the lake at a stone ramp, take a couple of minutes to walk down to the shore. Metallic structures at the far end make an intriguing photograph, especially in the mid-afternoon sun. Return up the stone path, turning into a small opening on a well-worn trail. A few steps in, the fully shaded forest opens up, with a creek on your right. Up the creek is a rock dam and a wall. Just past the wall is the earthen dam that forms the lake. Turn off the roadlike trail, rock-hop across the stream, and look for a large loblolly pine. Behind the pine is a step up to the wall and a path that leads to the top of the earthen dam. After crossing the dam, turn left for additional lakeside views.

Leaving the dam, the path curves right at 2.1 miles, following the shore of Arabia Lake, where it occasionally breaks into full sun. The metallic structures, which appear to be a unique type of pump, come into close range. Passing them on the right, the lake returns to a creek with extensive wetlands. At the north end of the wetlands, the narrow path curves right, crossing the wetlands in two places. This area may be impassible after a heavy rain. After the second muddy area, the path climbs a small knoll to a wooden bridge, still in full shade. At a three-way intersection at 2.5 miles, turn left and watch for a path on the right with a sign saying "Nature Center" and bearing an arrow; it's about 20 feet off to the right.

Now the path begins an extended, easy climb, crossing the multiuse trail and reentering the forest. As the footpath returns to the multiuse trail, follow it until you see a roadlike trail heading off on the right at 3.2 miles. Take this down to the three-way intersection, turn left, turn left on the multiuse trail, cross the bridge, and turn right, crossing Klondike Road. Follow the path until it turns to stone. You are standing between Bradley Mountain and Arabia Mountain. Directly in front of you and off to the right are two quarried ledges. The roads within the complex were used to haul stone back to the office, where it was weighed. Men were paid based on the amount of material quarried and the price of rock on the open market.

Turn around and return to the four-way intersection, then turn right. The road curves to the right, and the path returns to full sun as you walk out on the mountain. There are no cairns, but the path is easy to follow. (The path is about 20 to 30 feet to the right of the tree line that is at the bottom of Arabia Mountain.) When you approach a tree line, you'll easily spot the path through the trees. A large private lake on the left can be used to judge your location on the map. You'll see the cairns while you descend Bradley Mountain; follow them to the trail into the trees, where you will join the marked trail. Return along this path to your car.

NEARBY ATTRACTIONS

Both Stone Mountain (page 198) and Panola Mountain State Park (page 237) feature trails that climb to the top of similar rock structures

48 CHARLIE ELLIOTT WILDLIFE CENTER TRAILS

UTM Trailhead Coordinates

UTM Zone (NAD27) 17S

Easting 0246356

Northing 3706344

IN BRIEF

See a wide range of wildlife, including wild hogs, otters, beavers, deer, American bald eagles, and waterfowl on this relatively short hike.

DESCRIPTION

One of two parks under the management of Georgia's Wildlife Resources Division, the Charlie Elliott Wildlife Center is named for a local conservationist and educator who developed Georgia's State Park system and the Department of Natural Resources. Inside, a museum tells the life story of Charlie Elliott along an indoor hiking trail. His ashes were buried under a white pine that grows near the center.

This well-marked, well-maintained trail system is composed of four trails designated by the colors red (Clubhouse Trail), white (Pigeonhouse Trail), yellow (Murder Creek Trail), and blue (Granite Outcrop Trail). No hunting is allowed near these footpaths; however, hunting

----

Directions ————————————————→

From Atlanta take I-20 East to Exit 98 (Monticello/Mansfield). Turn right on GA 11 South. At 0.8 miles the road crosses US 278 at a four-way stop. Continue straight. At 4.3 miles there is a second four-way stop. Continue straight. At 9.5 miles turn left at the signed entrance to Charlie Elliott Wildlife Center (Marbin Farm Road). Travel 1.2 miles and turn right on Elliot Trail. In 0.6 miles turn left on an unnamed road at the Charlie Elliott Visitors Center sign. Park and walk toward the front entrance of the green-roofed visitor center. As you approach the museum, a path heads off to the right, marked by a brown hiker sign. Follow this 250 feet to a bulletin board. Look to the left for a red blaze to begin this hike.

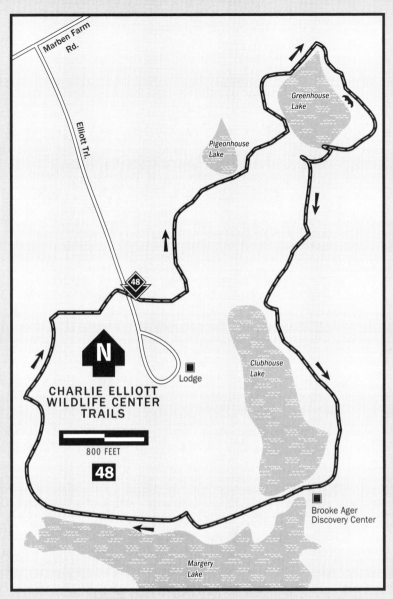

Marben Farm Rd.

Elliott Trl.

48

N

Lodge

**CHARLIE ELLIOTT
WILDLIFE CENTER
TRAILS**

800 FEET

48

*Pigeonhouse
Lake*

*Greenhouse
Lake*

*Clubhouse
Lake*

Brooke Ager
Discovery Center

*Margery
Lake*

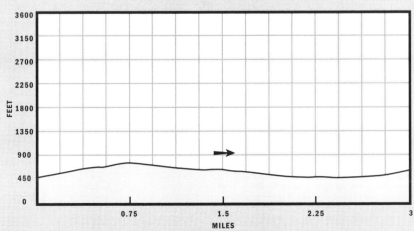

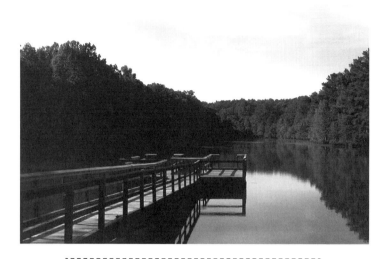

Dock on Clubhouse Lake at Charlie Elliott Wildlife Center

is permitted outside the safe zone. It is best to stay on the designated paths at all times. The hike begins in heavily shaded forest and makes an easy, steady climb to the trail's high point almost immediately. Toward the back of the visitor center, a man-made stream flows to a small pond. Passing the pond, the pathway curves left. Notice as you turn and climb that you can always see the next blaze. Near the top of the hill, there is a steep-sided valley on the right. In the center of the valley is an island of large granite boulders. On your left, slightly uphill, are more boulders.

At 0.2 miles, after a small bridge, bear left on the white (Pigeonhouse) trail, which begins a long, sweeping curve to the right, leading to Pigeonhouse and Greenhouse lakes. The footpath continues a slow, easy-paced rise between two ravines that run after a rain. As the trail nears the ridgetop, there is a small area for interpretive meetings off to the left. Shortly after the benches there is an old road, also off to the left. Three wooden walkovers in quick succession come at 0.3 miles, then there is a slightly longer gap before a fourth bridge.

Less than 50 feet past the last bridge, the trail suddenly emerges onto a manicured grass trail in full sun, with Pigeonhouse Lake to your left. There is a dock (fishing is allowed for designated groups only) slightly off the trail that affords an excellent viewing platform for bird-watchers. When approaching the lake, we flushed a blue heron, which flew off and circled some tall pines on the north side of the lake. Once convinced that we meant no harm, the heron returned, busily looking for fish. It is possible to see otters and beaver at all of the area lakes.

Turn around and walk straight ahead as you leave the dock. On the other side of the small parking area, pick up the white trail once again and turn left. At 0.6 miles a pathway heads off to the right, but continue straight ahead. Shortly after the intersection, the trail dips, and Greenhouse Lake comes into view. When the area was known as Preacher's Rock, this man-made lake was called Boyle

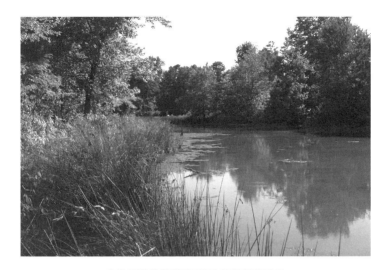

These lakes attract a lot of wildlife.

Lake Number One. You'll hear frequent loud firecracker-like pops of handguns and the rat-a-tat of small-arms fire from a firing range in the vicinity.

A century oak towers on the left side of the path, which begins to circle the lake. On the lake's north end, you enter the forest; the pathway makes a quick ascent and turns right. Quickly leaving the forest, the trail returns to full sun and manicured grass. After passing under power lines, the white trail bears right. Off to the right, a jetty extends past the shoreline for an excellent view of Greenhouse Lake at 0.8 miles. Coming off the jetty, turn right.

Circling the lake, you may spot an egret fishing, but your presence may cause the bird to relocate. Continue on this trail to a gazebo near the lakeshore. Walk past the gazebo on the lakeshore side and bear slightly left. Normally the trail is well blazed, but you'll encounter a short stretch of it where no white blazes are apparent. At the next intersection, bear right as the trail follows the water's edge. At 1.1 miles the pathway returns to shaded forest, and a few steps later there is a three-way intersection where all of the trails bear the white blaze. Take the path that runs by the lakeshore for a few feet to another dock for another opportunity to see waterfowl. As you leave the dock, turn left, return to the inter-section, and then turn right.

Over the next 1.5 miles, the trail is a mostly downhill affair in shaded forest, first following a creek to Clubhouse Lake then the lakeshore to Margery Lake. When you step across a creek at 1.3 miles, notice that tree sizes have increased, indicating an area of older growth. Look across the small gully ahead and to the right to see a wooden-slat ladder climbing to a hunter's stand. A tenth of a mile later, the white trail ends at the red (Clubhouse) trail. Turn left and continue on the red trail, which quickly curves to the right. Clubhouse Lake is on your right, shortly after the intersection.

From a distance the sound of croaking frogs fills the air. Side trails allow fisherfolk access from a low ridge, which the red trail follows. A bridge with stairs on each end, marks the hike's halfway point. After the bridge the trail moves away from the lake along an old roadbed, returning to Clubhouse Lake at the Brooke Ager Discovery Center. In addition to having an educational area, the center has picnic tables, restrooms, a small clubhouse, and a dock. There was a large number of crows (technically, a murder of crows) in the area when we hiked this trail, perhaps giving Murder Creek its name. Turn right and walk down a set of stairs and walk out on the dock.

Returning to the shore, turn right and cross an earthen embankment that impounds Clubhouse Lake. On the dam the trail becomes the yellow-blazed Murder Creek Trail. Note the significant difference in the levels of Clubhouse Lake (right) and Margery Lake (left). At the end of the embankment, the trail begins to zigzag, ending with a short climb as it becomes rocky and heavily rooted. In this area the pathway was loaded with spiderwebs, so duck under and around them when possible, or go with a group and volunteer to bring up the rear. Just shy of 2.5 miles, the trail turns right and begins an easy climb alongside Murder Creek. The cascading creek creates opportunities for photographers who aren't afraid to get their feet wet. At 2.8 miles the yellow trail reaches a T-intersection with the blue trail. Turn right on the blue trail, which begins as a narrow path on a level grassy plain then climbs toward the visitor center and the trailhead.

COCHRAN MILL TRAIL 49

IN BRIEF

After crossing Little Bear Creek, the trail follows an old road to Bear Creek, where it climbs along the riverbank to two falls. From the second falls, it rises to an old road and explores the Bear Creek watershed.

DESCRIPTION

Cochran Mill is one of those great hikes full of unexpected bonuses. Owen Henry Cochran inherited his father's land near Bear Creek and for many years ran a water-powered gristmill that his father had built. His brothers expanded the operation around the start of the 20th century. With the coming of electricity to rural Georgia, water power was no longer desirable, and the mill was abandoned. In the 1940s the land was used by the Klan for unknown purposes. Unfortunately, both mills were burned, and the dam to create the millrace was partially destroyed by vandals. A 48-foot-wide fieldstone dam built by Owen's brother remains. Fulton County built facilities on the 800-acre site, and in 1985 the privately funded Cochran Mill Nature Center was built beside the park.

KEY AT-A-GLANCE INFORMATION

LENGTH: 3 miles

CONFIGURATION: Loop

DIFFICULTY: Easy

SCENERY: 3 separate falls, large rock outcroppings and boulders

EXPOSURE: Full sun until you cross Bear Creek, then mostly shaded

TRAFFIC: Heavy to Bear Creek, moderate to the falls, then light

TRAIL SURFACE: Compacted dirt, portions on rock outcrops

HIKING TIME: 2 hours

ACCESS: Open year-round, dawn–dusk

MAPS: At Cochran Mill Nature Center, a privately run facility adjacent to the park; USGS Palmetto

FACILITIES: Restrooms, picnic tables at the entrance to the park; restrooms at the nature center

SPECIAL COMMENTS: Learn all about the history of the area, and its natural history, and view an assortment of animals at Cochran Mill Nature Center, through which the trail passes. There are separate trails for mountain-bike enthusiasts and equestrians. The Nature Center is open Monday through Saturday, 9 a.m. to 3 p.m.

Directions ⟶

Take I-85 South to Exit 56, Collingsworth Road (Palmetto/Tyrone). At the end of the ramp, turn right on Collingsworth Road. At 0.1 mile Collingsworth goes straight as Weldon Road heads off to the left. Collingsworth becomes Fayetteville Road. At a four-way stop at 2.4 miles, turn right on Toombs Street. Turn right on Hutchinson Ferry Road at 0.3 miles. Travel 1.4 miles and turn right on Cochran Mill Road. Travel 4.1 miles to the parking area on the left. Cochran Mill Nature Center is ahead on the right.

UTM Trailhead Coordinates

UTM Zone (NAD27) 16S

Easting   0712158

Northing   3716874

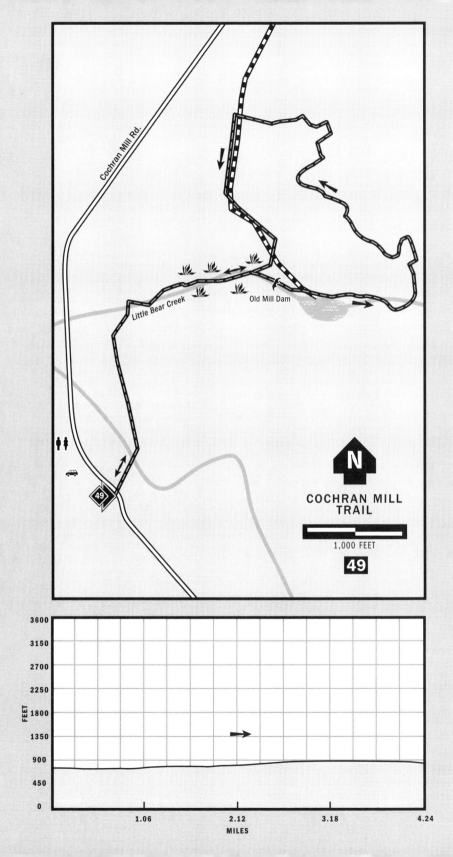

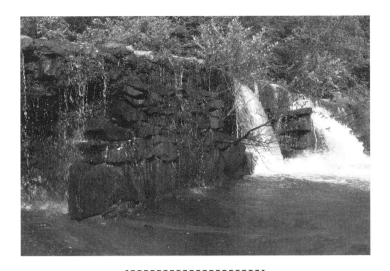

Old Mill Dam at Cochran Mill

From the parking lot, cross Cochran Mill Road, then follow the gravel road as it curves left and begins a moderate descent to Little Bear Creek. A concrete bridge has been sealed off to prevent people from using it, but carefully step down to the creek on the left side of the bridge. This is one we cross barefoot because it is deep and wide, ensuring wet feet.

As you cross the creek, watch on the right for the first of three falls along the hike. Put your shoes back on when you get to the far side of the creek because the grass is hard on bare feet. At the top of the hill near the bridge you'll have additional scenic views of the falls. From the bridge, travel straight ahead and down a level gravel road that takes you into a diverse hardwood forest. At 0.3 miles you'll find wild strawberries at the base of a large rock outcropping on the right. When the road comes to a fork 0.1 mile ahead, take the road on the right and continue to a second bridge, this one over Bear Creek. A cleverly arranged entrance is designed to be wide enough for a human but too narrow for bikes and horses. After crossing the bridge, turn right and begin to climb in full shade at an easy-to-moderate grade along the bank of Bear Creek.

If you watch closely, you will see an old yellow blaze every once in a while, but don't worry if you don't see it. Except in a couple of places on rock outcroppings, the trail is well worn and easy to follow. One of these comes quickly at 0.7 miles into the hike. Keep the river and falls on your right and climb until the trail enters the woods, still near the stream's bank. As you reenter the full shade of the forest, there is an area of perma-mud. At 0.8 miles the trail splits; bear right—the other path is the return from the loop. Following the split the footpath begins to make a significant moderate climb.

Watch for the destroyed dam on the right; water emerges on the left, falls a few feet, and slides back to the right. Not much else remains of Owen Cochran's mill. As you climb the rock outcropping, you will see a large stone with a square center cutout. It marks the path, which rises to a level road with an embankment on the left. Still following the creek, the trail begins to curve left at 1.2 miles. At the curve, watch for an excellent view of wetlands in the distance.

Climbing into the watershed of Bear Creek on a moderate grade, you'll reach the top of an unnamed knoll. The trail then falls to a small creek, which it crosses on a wooden plank bridge with no railings. After the bridge the trail bears right and begins to climb the next knoll. Just before the top, the path makes a left-hand turn, then descends to Cochran Mills Nature Center. Entering from the back, you will pass a large iguana and other animals before coming to the wooden building. We stopped and talked with Rick McCarthy and Cory Washington, who were very helpful, especially with area history, and we got to spend time with some unique creatures.

With the pond on your right, walk along a gravel road to a trailhead kiosk off the road on the left. Follow the path as it descends to a left turn at 2.1 miles. About 0.2 miles later, bear right at a three-way intersection and continue to the right when the trail crosses a stone outcrop to return you to the middle falls of Bear Creek on your left. Continue along this trail back to your car.

NEARBY ATTRACTIONS

From mid-April to the first week in June, the Georgia Renaissance Festival takes visitors to Renaissance Europe. Performers such as the Tortuga Twins and the Zucchini Brothers (Ripe and Green) entertain the masses until it's time for the jousts. The event is held weekends, including Memorial Day, from 10:30 a.m. to 6 p.m.

HIGH FALLS TRAIL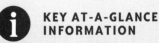

IN BRIEF

This trail explores High Falls State Park, including the waterfalls on the Towaliga River and a mill and sluice.

DESCRIPTION

From the overlook, look just right of the modern road to the remains of a gristmill. Built before the Civil War on the Old Alabama Road, the mill had attracted a small community by 1860. Confederate troops burned the mill as Union troops advanced toward it during Sherman's March to the Sea. Following the Civil War, the mill was rebuilt, and the town once again began to grow. In addition to the gristmill, there was a post office, cotton mill, factories, and a blacksmith shop. A major east–west connector, the Alabama Road gave the settlers the means to transport their goods.

Once known as Unionville, the city was called High Falls after the Civil War. According to local legends, Towaliga means "roasted scalp" in Creek, but the most probable translation is "sumac place." Construction on the dam to the right was begun in 1890 by the Towaliga Falls Power Company. Shortly thereafter the city found out that the railroad was passing them by. Many residents decided to follow the railroad to Jackson, and work on

KEY AT-A-GLANCE INFORMATION

LENGTH: 2.2 miles

CONFIGURATION: Loop

DIFFICULTY: Moderate

SCENERY: Cascades and waterfalls along Towaliga Creek

EXPOSURE: Full sun near the dam, partial sun to full shade elsewhere

TRAFFIC: Heavy on the Falls Trail, light elsewhere

TRAIL SURFACE: Packed dirt

HIKING TIME: 1.5 hours

ACCESS: Closed Mondays, except major holidays

MAPS: Handout at kiosk; USGS High Falls

FACILITIES: Swimming area, picnic tables, restrooms

SPECIAL COMMENTS: There are many additional outdoor activities at this state park close to I-75, including boating, swimming, fishing, and miniature golf.

Directions

Take I-75 South to Exit 198, High Falls Road. At the end of the ramp, turn left (there is no traffic light). At 1.6 miles, turn into the second entrance on the left, just after crossing a bridge. After paying a $3 parking fee at the entrance kiosk, find a parking spot on the left side of the road and return to the overlook to the right of the kiosk, where the trail narrative begins.

UTM Trailhead Coordinates

UTM Zone (NAD27) 16S

Easting 0778036

Northing 3674965

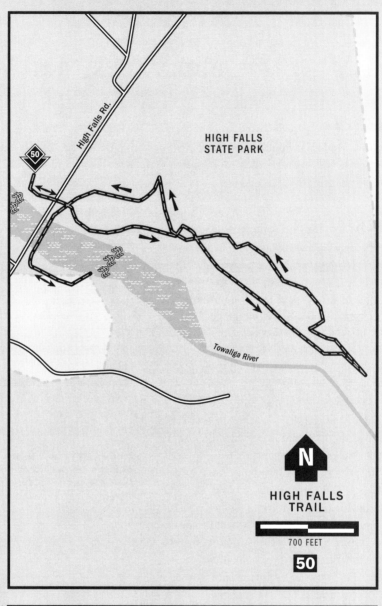

HIGH FALLS
STATE PARK

High Falls Rd.

50

Towaliga River

N

HIGH FALLS
TRAIL

700 FEET

50

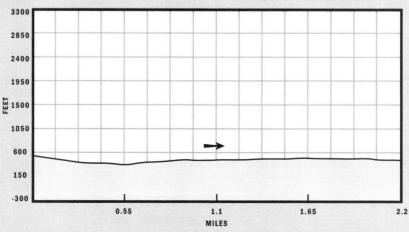

3300
2850
2400
1950
1500
1050
600
150
-300

FEET

0.55   1.1   1.65   2.2
MILES

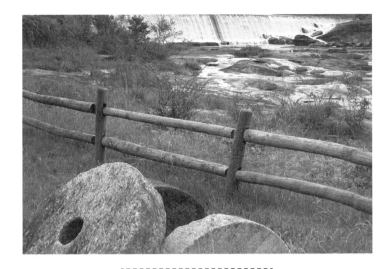

Historic millstones at High Falls

the dam came to a halt. In 1905 the property was sold to the Georgia Hydro-Electric Company, which completed the dam.

In 1902 a steel bridge was completed that spanned Towaliga Creek above the falls. The remains of the bridge are still visible. Flooding that followed Hurricane Alberto in 1994 brought so much debris down the river that the supports for a portion of the bridge were destroyed, and the bridge collapsed. From the overlook follow the road past the kiosk and cross the street, stepping up to a deck-like structure on the far side of the road. This is the trailhead for both High Falls Nature Trail and Falls Trail. Walk past the nature trail on the left down to the signed entrance to Falls Trail on the right. Descend a set of alternating wooden steps and boardwalk until the trail turns left at the end of the boardwalk and runs near the bank of the river. The compacted-soil trail is covered with gravel to help with footing in this moist environment. Finally, at 0.2 miles, the view opens up, and Towaliga River becomes a series of cascades and falls on the right as the water playfully darts between and over large boulders in the river. In the center, the 20-to 30-foot drop is the falls' largest.

The red-blazed trail parallels the river but does not run adjacent to it at all times. Trails off to the right provide access for fishing or for a better view of the falls. Trails to the left allow hikers to explore the river's small floodplain. The mixed second-growth piedmont forest is composed of American beech, shortleaf pine, and hemlock. At just over 0.3 miles the trail turns left, quickly approaching a confusing intersection at a bridge as it follows a tributary upstream. Turn right and cross the bridge, then turn right again. Ignore the red blazes straight ahead at the bridge; they are for the return trail, which also uses this bridge. A four-way trail intersection just past the bridge may also be confusing. Continue straight ahead.

Running some 20 feet above the river, the trail now offers occasional long-distance scenic views, especially in winter and early spring. Boulders are scattered about here, with some impressive rock outcroppings that combine to create something of a maze, which the kids should love. Watch for the blazes and follow the well-worn trail where there are none. Don't get discouraged by the lack of blazes; we were about to turn around when a red blaze suddenly appeared high on a tree.

Climbing away from the river, a switchback eases the rise. Near the top of the hill, turn right where the trail reaches a three-way intersection. Now the trail begins to undulate, becomes rockier, and follows the curves of the hills as it runs some 60 feet above Towaliga Creek. A boulder-strewn tributary at 0.8 miles makes for a good photo opportunity, but you will need a tripod and long exposure time to shoot it because a heavy canopy of trees limits the light. At 1 mile the trail makes a hard left turn. A few feet ahead, a wooden bridge spans another scenic creek. After crossing the bridge, the trail turns right and begins a rapid ascent, curving back around to the left. The wooden bridge is now down a steep embankment on your left as the trail slowly comes around to the right. Crossing the outgoing trail, the path comes to the confusing bridge, and the markings are now easy to understand. Cross the bridge and turn right, following the path as it climbs a ridge.

A few feet past a double blaze, the footpath makes a hard left and joins High Falls Nature Trail. An unblazed trail appears to continue straight ahead, but it quickly ends. According to the High Falls map, the blaze on the nature trail is white, but it seems to have a yellowish tint; there are red blazes as well. On returning to the deck, turn right, then turn left and cross the bridge. Turn right at the Historic Trail sign. Almost immediately on the right is a sluice that powered an electric plant farther down the river. This plant supplied power to area businesses from 1905 until 1958, when it closed after 53 years of service. Georgia Power transferred the plant and some adjoining land to the Hiawassee Timber Company, which gave it to the State of Georgia in 1966.

On the left, 1.7 miles into the hike, a trail departs at a 45-degree angle. Follow this down to an overlook that affords an excellent view of High Falls. Return to the historic trail and continue down to a gated dam used to control water flow to the power plant. Turn around and return to the road.

NEARBY ATTRACTIONS

Fresh Air Barbecue in Jackson has been serving Georgia-style barbecue since 1929 and is generally recognized as the best in the state. Find them on GA 42/US 23; phone (770) 775-3182.

MCINTOSH RESERVE TRAIL 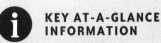 51

IN BRIEF

The trail explores the banks of the Chattahoochee River, then turns inland and climbs to check out the adjacent watershed.

DESCRIPTION

Creek chief William McIntosh was the son of Captain William McIntosh of the Georgia militia and a Creek woman. When the United States declared war in 1813 on a faction of the Creek Nation known as the Red Sticks, McIntosh joined Andrew Jackson and led Creek warriors against the Red Sticks. Despite McIntosh's leading a majority of the Creek Nation against this violent faction, Jackson demanded millions of acres of land from the tribe.

McIntosh's cousin, George Troup, advanced a political platform that included removal of the Creek during his successful bid for governor of Georgia in 1823. In 1825 McIntosh signed the Treaty of Indian Springs, which relinquished control of much of the remaining Creek land in Georgia. When the Creek found out that part of the treaty included

---

Directions

Take I-85 South to Exit 37/GA 34 (Newnan, Shenandoah). At the end of the ramp, turn right on Bullsboro Drive (GA 34). In 0.2 miles turn right on West Bypass 34 at the KFC and Gold's Gym. At 4.5 miles turn right on GA 16/North Alternate 27. At 8.6 miles turn left on north GA 5 in downtown Whitesburg at the Citgo Station. Travel 2.3 miles, turning left at the sign for McIntosh Reserve. At 1.6 miles register at the Ranger Station and pay the $2 fee. The road passes the McIntosh homestead, which is also the site of the Creek chief's grave. At the end of the road, there is a parking lot on the left.

---

i KEY AT-A-GLANCE INFORMATION

LENGTH: 5.9 miles

CONFIGURATION: Loop

DIFFICULTY: Moderate

SCENERY: Chattahoochee River views from the riverbank and nearby hills, extensive forested wetlands, pond created by beaver dam, historic building

EXPOSURE: Full sun in the Chattahoochee floodplain, mostly shaded as the trail climbs into the watershed

TRAFFIC: Light

TRAIL SURFACE: Compacted dirt, some gravel roads

HIKING TIME: 2.5 hours

ACCESS: Daily, 8 a.m.–dusk; closed Thanksgiving, December 25, and January 1

MAPS: Available at park ranger office; USGS Whitesburg

FACILITIES: Restrooms at trailhead and in a play area about two-thirds of the way through the trail; picnic tables, playground

SPECIAL COMMENTS: On the road to the trailhead are the homestead and grave of William McIntosh. The first home was burned by the Creek Indians on the night they murdered Chief McIntosh. A similar home and tavern were later moved to this site.

UTM Trailhead Coordinates

UTM Zone (NAD27) 16S

Easting   0690366

Northing   3702016

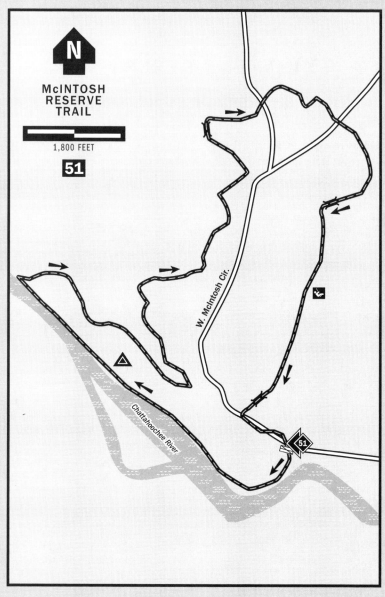

N

McINTOSH
RESERVE
TRAIL

1,800 FEET

51

W. McIntosh Cir.

Chattahoochee River

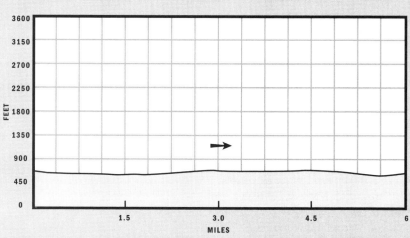

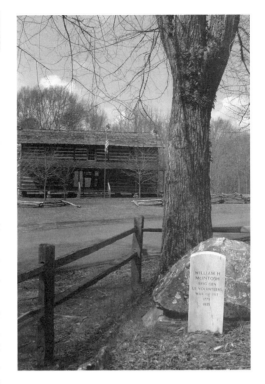

Grave of William McIntosh in front of homestead

McIntosh's receiving a plantation on the Chattahoochee River, a supporter of the Red Sticks led a raid, in which they killed McIntosh.

Beginning as a gravel roadbed to the right of the restrooms, the trail turns right at a brown gate and falls quickly to a 90-degree turn in the Chattahoochee River. Here, you'll enjoy an excellent view of the river as it flows south. The footpath turns right and follows the river past an overlook in the picnic area atop a rock bluff. The fast-flowing Chattahoochee River has ample floodplains, which this hike explores during the first 1.3 miles. These broad floodplains, which extend up to 0.5 miles wide in the area, are much larger than the floodplains of the Chattahoochee River National Recreation Area parks farther north. Their size reflects the river's growing power as it flows south. For many miles, small tributaries, such as the one bridged at 0.4 miles, have joined the river as it flows to the southwest corner of Georgia.

A series of rock outcroppings at 0.6 miles extends into the riverbed as a shoal. Just past the outcropping is a sign instructing hikers to keep off the riverbank just before the footpath juts inland slightly. Stately oak, elm, and beech struggle to stabilize the riverbank in an area of picnic tables and grills. At 0.9 miles the picnic area is replaced by an open field designed for a variety of sports, including flying radio-controlled airplanes.

Continuing in full sun, the footpath turns left at 1.4 miles and follows the shore of an extensive forested wetland (identified as a beaver pond on the map) as it slowly curves to the right. Coming off to the left at 1.5 miles, a side trail briefly explores the low pond. The footpath makes a U-turn at the end of the pond as it continues to follow the edge, then quickly makes a second U-turn before it begins to climb into the watershed of the Chattahoochee River. The trail turns left at a cut in the rocks and descends to an old railroad bed, which it leaves at 2.4 miles to enter a forest of oak, beech, and pine.

McIntosh Reserve Trail now begins a steady climb as it makes a sweeping curve to the right around a tall knoll. At 2.7 miles the trail splits. Take the trail that bears left; it comes to a boundary marker running along a dirt road that marks the edge of the park. The trail soon turns right, back into the park. When you come to a yellow-blazed trail, turn left. Note the trees on the right with embedded barbed wire. In this area the trail is being heavily reworked, but the new trail, marked with detour signs, is easy to follow.

Crossing a bridge over a stream at 3.5 miles, the trail climbs to an old roadbed, which it follows to a detour sign before leading to a trail that climbs into the woods. After crossing a gravel road at 3.8 miles, the trail levels then begins a moderate climb to its high point at 4.1 miles, where it crosses the paved road into the park. From this point the trail falls at an easy-to-moderate grade, reaching a wet-foot stream crossing at 4.5 miles, then turning right and climbing a hill as the trail curves around to the left. Less than 0.1 mile later, a trail branches off to the right, but continue straight ahead. Numerous wooden platforms in the area indicate this was once a developed campsite. A second trail, off to the right at 4.8 miles, leads to a trash dump.

From this point the trail enters full sun in an open field. As you enter an area with a children's playground and restrooms, watch the bushes on the left side of the field for an opening that leads to a wide-stream crossing. Take a few steps to the right, where the river is easier to cross. After crossing, turn right and follow the trail as it winds through the floodplain. Occasionally the trail splits, almost always to avoid a wet area. At 5.5 miles the trail crosses the stream on a wooden bridge and then turns left on the paved park road.

NEARBY ATTRACTIONS

Coweta County Courthouse, in downtown Newnan on Alternate 27, was built in 1903. The tower reaches 100 feet and dominates the county seat, which is country-music star Alan Jackson's hometown.

OCMULGEE RIVER TRAIL   52

IN BRIEF

The trail parallels the Ocmulgee River along its floodplain, occasionally moving inland to circumvent a tributary or marshy area.

DESCRIPTION

Ocmulgee, meaning bubbling water or boiling water, is the name that was given to this strong, wide river by the Hitchiti tribe. Early British explorers knew it as the Ocheese Creek and called the native people living along the river near present-day Macon the Creek. The Hitchiti was one nation within the Creek Confederacy. It is believed, but cannot be proven, that the Creek were the descendants of Mound Builders who built cities near the confluence of two or more rivers throughout Georgia. Ocmulgee, Etowah, and Kolomoki mounds are all examples of the work of America's first tribal civilization in Georgia.

As we pulled into the Oconee National Forest parking area, a family of wild turkeys hurried away from the rear of the parking area, so watch out for wildlife throughout the hike. Ocmulgee River Trail begins by rising through the forest and quickly beginning an easy, even descent toward the river on a wide, roadlike path. Throughout most of the hike, the trail is

KEY AT-A-GLANCE INFORMATION

LENGTH: 5.2 miles
CONFIGURATION: Out-and-back
DIFFICULTY: Easy
SCENERY: Ocmulgee River floodplain, some good views of the Ocmulgee River
EXPOSURE: Some sun
TRAFFIC: Light
TRAIL SURFACE: Packed dirt
HIKING TIME: 2 hours
ACCESS: Open year-round
MAPS: Berner
FACILITIES: None
SPECIAL COMMENTS: The footpath now continues to the Ocmulgee River bluffs, about 16 miles from the trailhead.

Directions

Take I-75 South from Atlanta to exit 187 (GA 83/Forsyth/Montecello). Turn left on SR 83, known locally as North Lee Street and Cabaniss Road. The highway crosses US 23 and begins a descent to the Ocmulgee River. After crossing the river on a double bridge, the road begins to rise. Watch on the left for an unmarked pulloff big enough for five or six cars. The trailhead is on the river side of the parking lot, near the highway, on top of a small mound.

UTM Trailhead Coordinates

UTM Zone (NAD27) 16S
Easting   0741854
Northing   3736068

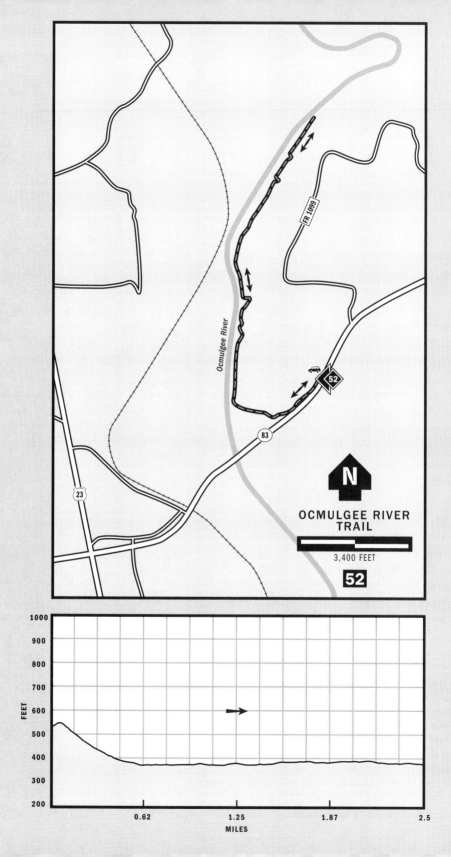

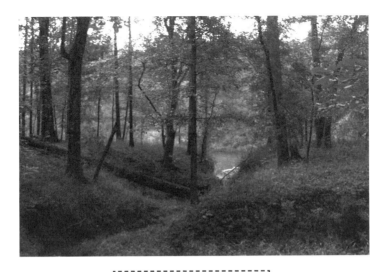

Tributary to the Ocmulgee River

wide, narrowing occasionally to cross a stream or swampy area, making this a good family hike. After dropping 200 feet in 0.6 miles, the trail reaches the Ocmulgee River and easily curves to the right to parallel the wide, fast-flowing watercourse. Throughout the hike the Ocmulgee will be on your left on the way out, and on your right on the way back. Car noise quickly disappears as you walk away from GA 83 along the riverbank. From here on, watch carefully for poison ivy.

You occasionally have long-distance views from the trail, and there are oaks and elms along the path. Many of the elms are large and have deep furrows and ashen-gray bark, indicating they are fairly old. These elm trees, along with substantial oaks, anchor the healthy riparian zones on either side of the river. The U.S. Forest Service, which manages the area, permits horseback riding on the trail. During our hike we noticed evidence of horses and spotted a number of fairly common birds and wildlife, including wood ducks, vireos, squirrels, deer, and raccoons. Since the river is along their migration path, large numbers of waterfowl can be spotted during the spring and fall.

As the trail comes to the first tributary of the Ocmulgee, it bears right (inland), making a wet-foot crossing of a stream at just under 1 mile. The trail climbs away from the river again at 1.2 miles, crossing a wooden bridge without rails, and climbs to a primitive camping area at 1.3 miles. You can walk through the camping area to a small forest service parking area or simply make a hard left at the start of the primitive camping area. On the trail's return to the Ocmulgee the river traverses a swampy area before climbing to the riverbank 0.1 mile later. From here the trail follows the riverbank closely, only occasionally dropping into the lightly forested floodplain. At 2.6 miles the trail turns inland to cross another stream. Although we could see that the trail continues, this looked like a good place to turn around and head back to the car.

NEARBY ATTRACTIONS

The Ocmulgee River flows south to Macon, where it passes through the Ocmulgee National Monument, an Early Mississippian Mound Builder site that flourished between 900 and 1150 AD. Within the park grounds are a museum and several larger mounds that are fun to climb. To get there, return to I-75 south and take Exit 165; follow the signs to I-16. Take Exit 2 and turn left on Coliseum Drive. In 0.6 miles turn right on Emery Highway. Follow this 0.8 miles. The entrance is on the right.

PANOLA MOUNTAIN TRAIL 53

IN BRIEF

Two interpreted loop trails take hikers though two very different environments; the first trail drops to a creek that is occasionally dry, while the second climbs one of Panola Mountain's many outcroppings.

DESCRIPTION

Panola Mountain State Conservation Park was established in 1971 and is Georgia's first "conservation park." Located on a massive granite rock outcrop, its job is to protect many of the environmentally sensitive areas within the park, both biologic and geologic, on this 100-acre monadnock (single mountain). The trails within the park are individual loops, and the only developed side trails take visitors to interpreted areas. The trails involve less than a 150-foot elevation change, with the greatest part of that on Watershed Trail.

Exiting the nature center, continue to a large trailhead sign and turn right. After passing through a pine blowdown with evidence of a fire, Watershed Trail begins an easy descent as it enters a fertile piedmont lowlands with hickory, oak, and sumac. The trail is wide and strewn with wood chips, but it changes to a dirt trail as it drops at an easy grade to a three-way intersection. Continue straight ahead, in

KEY AT-A-GLANCE INFORMATION

LENGTH: 3.3 miles (including a 1-mile fitness path)

CONFIGURATION: Double loop

DIFFICULTY: Easy

SCENERY: Some good long-distance views from rock outcropping

EXPOSURE: Much of the trail is full sun.

TRAFFIC: Moderate, especially on weekends

TRAIL SURFACE: Mostly dirt but some stone

HIKING TIME: 1.5 hours

ACCESS: Open year-round, $4 park entrance fee

MAPS: Interpreted trail maps are available at the trailhead kiosk; USGS Stockbridge, Redan.

FACILITIES: Natural history exhibits; interpreted trails; restrooms

SPECIAL COMMENTS: A ranger-led hike on the third Saturday of the month explores environmentally sensitive Panola Mountain. Call beforehand to be certain the hike is scheduled and to reserve a spot.

Directions ⟶

From Atlanta, take I-20 East to Exit 68, Wesley Chapel Road. Turn right and, at 0.3 miles, turn left at a traffic light, onto Snapfinger Road. The entrance to the park is 5.8 miles on the left. Continue to the end of the road, enter the nature center, , and pick up two pamphlets, one for Watershed Trail and one for Rock Outcrop Trail.

UTM Trailhead Coordinates

UTM Zone (NAD27) 16S

Easting 0741854

Northing 3736068

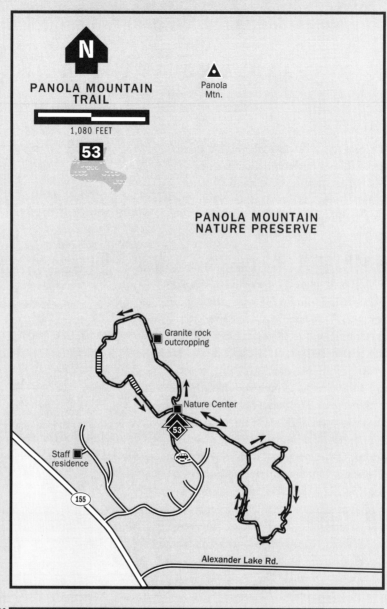

PANOLA MOUNTAIN TRAIL

N

△ Panola Mtn.

1,080 FEET

53

PANOLA MOUNTAIN NATURE PRESERVE

Granite rock outcropping

Nature Center

53

Staff residence

155

Alexander Lake Rd.

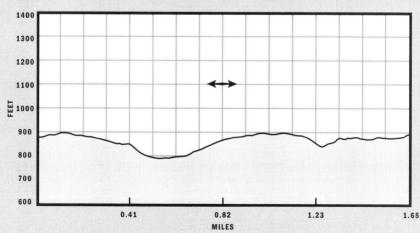

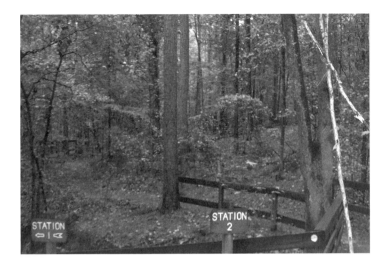

Interpreted watershed trail

the direction the pamphlet describes, to reach a creek. Watch for streams that carry watershed runoff down to the creek, shaping the landscape as they go—the path crosses two of these on bridges. The first station leaves the trail to take hikers to a small gully created by erosion.

Stations 2 and 3 continue the hydrology lesson, but Station 4 takes hikers out to a flat "pavement rock" formed by an exfoliation process enhanced by the creek water. Finally, the interpretive stations introduce hikers to lichen, a plant that grows on exposed granite to create an environment where some plants, especially red moss, may follow. Cross another bridge and begin climbing back into the watershed of the stream. As the loop trail comes to a T-intersection at 0.8 miles, turn right and return to the trailhead.

At the trailhead, turn right again and follow Rock Outcrop Trail. This trail traverses a vastly different environment than Watershed Trail, circling a low hill with surprising drops off to right and a thicker forest to the left. The tree mix has also changed, with loblolly pine, sweetgum, black cherry, and hawthorn accenting white oak on this yellow-blazed trail. The trail begins to descend when you see the first of the massive granite outcrops at 1.2 miles. Less than 0.1 mile later, this hike passes rock cairns; a single pole rail keeps visitors on the proper path. Because of the sensitive environment, please stay on the hiking trail and don't be tempted to stray. If you would like to spend time on similar slabs, see Arabia Mountain Trail (page 212) or the Stone Mountain Historic Trail Stone Mountain Loop (page 193), or Stone Mountain Mountaintop Trail (page 198). A small portion of the trail does traverse the granite.

After viewing the granite, continue to two boardwalks—one to the right, the other to the left—that take you to the trail interpretation. There is a small outdoor theater on the left before you reach the trailhead kiosk.

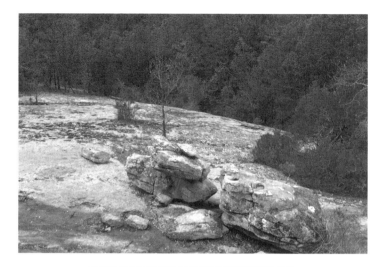

Rock outcrop along trail of the same name

If you decide to make the ranger-led trek to Panola Mountain, be certain to wear comfortable hiking shoes. The loop hike travels 3.5 miles to the largest exposed granite slab in the park and back again, and you'll stop frequently to discuss various topics.

NEARBY ATTRACTIONS

Continue south on GA 155 to McDonough, turn left on John Frank Ward Boulevard, then turn right on Lemon Street and proceed to GA 81. Turn left on Lake Dow Road and enter Heritage Park. Baseball fields occupy most of the park, but it does have a 0.9-mile multiuse track and a heritage area that's worth the visit. The park is open 8 a.m.–11 p.m. and features a covered bridge and a veteran's memorial. A visit to the heritage museum requires you make an appointment; phone (770) 288-8421.

PEACHTREE CITY CART PATH 54

IN BRIEF

This hike explores Flat Creek, which creates Lake Peachtree, and a forested wetlands south of the dam. On the return trip, you visit city hall and cross GA 54 on an impressive pedestrian overpass.

DESCRIPTION

Embroiled in battles over integration, hardly anybody in Atlanta seemed to notice when bulldozers began sculpting a little corner of land 25 miles south of the city in rural Fayette County. The Phipps family (for whom Phipps Plaza was later named) and their New York–based investment company, Bessemer Properties, purchased thousands of acres of farmland and began building streets, houses, and golf courses in the 1950s. The cart path was a logical extension of the concept and today affords visitors and residents almost 90 miles of multiuse paths.

Lake Kedron, where the hike begins, is a 235-acre lake owned by the Fayette County water system. The large public parking area connects to the Peachtree City cart path at the south end of the park across Interlochen Drive. Initially climbing through a majority pine (mostly loblolly) forest, commonly found south of Atlanta, the cart path parallels Peachtree Parkway as it climbs to Walt Banks

KEY AT-A-GLANCE INFORMATION

LENGTH: 11.3 miles
CONFIGURATION: Loop
DIFFICULTY: Moderate
SCENERY: Lakeside views, forested wetlands, mansions
EXPOSURE: Mostly full sun, except in the area of Flat Creek Nature Center
TRAFFIC: Heavy
TRAIL SURFACE: Asphalt, some wood and compacted soil
HIKING TIME: 5.5 hours
ACCESS: Open year-round, dawn–dusk
MAPS: Peachtree City Holiday Inn and many other businesses; USGS Tyrone
FACILITIES: Restrooms in parks, including at Kedron Lake trailhead; picnic tables, some with grills; playgrounds along the hike
SPECIAL COMMENTS: The cart path is a multiuse trail that allows electric golf carts. Kids are permitted to drive carts in Peachtree City. The hike's strategically located parks with playgrounds are great for the kids.

Directions

Take I-85 South to Exit 61, Fairburn, GA 74/ Senoia Road. At the end of the ramp, turn left and travel 7.4 miles to Peachtree Parkway. Turn left at the light and travel 1.8 miles to Fayette County's Lake Kedron Park and Reservoir on the left. Enter the parking lot and continue to the far end.

UTM Trailhead Coordinates

UTM Zone (NAD27) 16S

Easting   0725970

Northing   3700631

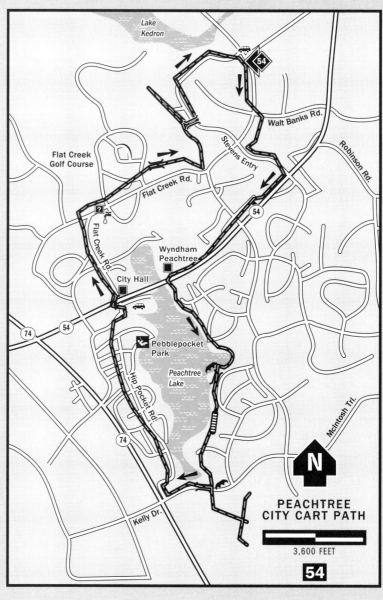

PEACHTREE CITY CART PATH

3,600 FEET

54

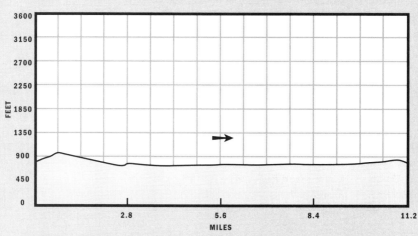

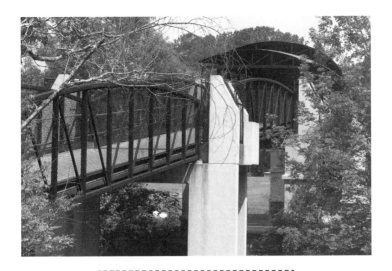

Pedestrian overpass across Floy Farr Road

Road, which it crosses at 0.5 miles, before turning left. After crossing Peachtree Parkway, the cart path parallels Walt Banks Road to a four-way intersection, where the cart path turns left before an unsigned road and begins an easy climb.

Just over 1 mile into the hike, the path turns right, crosses this road, then turns left, continuing to run next to the road as it levels off. At GA 54, also known as Floy Farr Parkway, the cart path makes a hard right. Farr, a Tyrone banker, provided much of the funding for the development of Peachtree City, and he and his family were deeply involved in Fayette County politics.

Dropping to a three-way intersection where the trail reaches a T-intersection, turn right (there is a tunnel to the left). This path quickly curves left and abruptly comes out at a McDonald's, which is on the left. On the right is Peachtree Pointe shopping center, a strip mall featuring Bicycles Unlimited, Wild Birds Unlimited, and Yoshi's Dog House. Walk to North Peachtree Parkway, cross the road, and continue straight, past a day care center and church. At the far end of the church parking lot, rejoin the cart path, turning left at 1.7 miles as you step onto the path, which almost immediately curves right.

Honeysuckle and Virginia creeper fill a white oak and loblolly pine forest that approaches old-growth size as the trail drops into a vale adjacent to but beneath GA 54. Coming into full sun, the path drops into a gully formed by the road's embankment and a parking lot, before crossing the entrance to the Wyndham Peachtree Hotel and Conference Center. After the road the path drops, quickly curving left and joining what appears to be a wide creek as it passes under Floy Farr Parkway. At 2.3 miles the path curves left again as Lake Peachtree suddenly opens up before you in a scenic long-distance view down the lake. Continue a few feet to a four-way intersection and turn left. The cart path rises and curves left to a bridge for a better view of the lake. Return to the four-way intersection and go straight as the path follows the lakeshore, with upscale homes on the right. Asphalt paths to the left allow access to the lake from nearby roads.

The cart path jogs right, then left, at 2.8 miles. After the jog there is a fishing dock on the right, and the path crosses between two lakes on an earthen dam before reaching Battery Way Boat Dock. At 3.4 miles the path curves right, continuing along the lakeshore as a couple of paths join from the left. The path turns right at a split-rail fence when it climbs away from the lake in an area with homes on either side. At 4.1 miles the cart path crosses a paved road, McIntosh Trail. Disregard a sign pointing left to the nature center and continue along the cart path to a wooden boardwalk at 4.8 miles. Turn left at the boardwalk, crossing a forested wetland with a more diverse forest of sweetgum, black gum, water oak, and pignut hickory joining the standard hardwood mix.

When the boardwalk ends, a compacted-soil trail explores a knoll with a garden featuring many native plants. In this area are an amphitheater, city administration buildings, and a BMX track. Return to the cart path, cross it, and continue to the boardwalk on the other side. This section of the boardwalk explores the creek, curving south and running alongside the bank. Return to the cart path, turn left, cross McIntosh Trail, and turn left again. At the bridge Flat Creek flows out of Lake Peachtree as a spillway.

Follow the markings as the cart path crosses McIntosh Trail, continues a few yards, and crosses McIntosh again at 5.9 miles, this time at Hip Pocket Road. Over the next 1.3 miles, the trail closely follows this suburban road, occasionally sharing a well-marked track with vehicular traffic. At 7.1 miles Pebblepocket Park offers swings, slides, and other equipment, including a rock-climbing wall and picnic tables. Make the next left at Willow Bend, and on the right you'll see Memorial Park, dedicated to a local resident who was 17 when she died. Just beyond the park is a second playground, then the cart path enters a parking lot. Look on the far side for a bridge; cross it and turn left, then right, and the cart path is directly in front of you. At city hall the path turns right, along Floy Farr Parkway. A fountain at 7.5 miles makes a good rest stop.

Retrace your steps to Willow Bend, cross, and continue past a church on the left and an open space known as the Village Green on the right. Watch for the crossover bridge on the right and head for it when the path reaches an intersection. After crossing, turn right at the four-way intersection. This path follows Floy Farr Parkway and then curves left, following Flat Creek Road until it crosses two streets in quick succession. At the T-intersection, turn right. The trail drops to Flat Creek, which has been developed into a golf course. As the path rises, watch for the impressive clubhouse on the left, across the street. After the course the path turns left at a four-way intersection.

Entering full shade the path comes to a bridge at 10.1 miles, across Flat Creek. On the right are some lovely cascades and falls as the creek comes out of Lake Kedron. Turn around and take any of the first three paths to the left to return to Interlochen Drive. Turn left and follow the road around to Lake Kedron Park.

NEARBY ATTRACTIONS

Peachtree City is the home to the Atlanta area weather forecasting office. Located at Falcon Field they offer one-hour tours of the facility to groups, families, and individuals, Monday through Friday at 10 a.m. and 1 p.m. During times of inclement weather the tours are canceled. To schedule a tour, contact the Administrative Assistant at (770) 486-1133 ext. 221. She will call you back with a confirmed tour date and time. Adult-to-child ratios are strictly enforced. Tours last about one hour. The National Weather Service office is located at 4 Falcon Drive, Peachtree City 30269. To get there, take I-85 south to Exit 61 (Fairburn and Peachtree City). From the Exit 61 off-ramp, make a left turn onto GA 74 South. It is a 10-mile, 20-minute drive to the facility. At the intersection of GA 74 and Crosstown/TDK, make a right turn onto TDK Boulevard, then a left turn at the stop sign onto Dividend Road. Take a right turn onto Falcon Field. Enter the first building on the left.

55 PIEDMONT NATIONAL WILDLIFE REFUGE TRAILS

KEY AT-A-GLANCE INFORMATION

LENGTH: 3.8 miles

CONFIGURATION: Double loop

DIFFICULTY: Easy

SCENERY: Lakeside and creekside views and forested wetlands

EXPOSURE: Full sun in the vicinity of Allison Lake and the dam; mostly sunny on Red-Cockaded Woodpecker Trail; mostly shaded on Allison Lake Trail, except near the lakeshore

TRAFFIC: Light

TRAIL SURFACE: Compacted dirt trails, gravel roads

HIKING TIME: 2 hours

ACCESS: Open year-round

MAPS: Available at trailhead kiosk; USGS Dames Ferry

FACILITIES: Visitor center on the road is open Monday–Friday, 8 a.m.–5 p.m.

SPECIAL COMMENTS: This is an excellent trail for bird-watchers and wildlife lovers, but be wary of ticks and chiggers.

UTM Trailhead Coordinates

UTM Zone (NAD27) 17S

Easting 0249492

Northing 3666963

IN BRIEF

This hike combines Red-Cockaded Woodpecker Trail and Allison Lake to take you through a wilderness rich with wildlife.

DESCRIPTION

Our introduction to Piedmont National Wildlife Refuge was certainly thrilling. A black vulture with a wingspan as wide as the road led us to the trailhead, finally rising above the tree line and turning away from Allison Lake. Ringed in fieldstone with a dark brown roof, the trailhead kiosk contains extensive information on the creation and goals of Piedmont NWR and the National Wildlife Refuge Program in general. You'll also find information on the preservation of species native to the park, including the endangered red-cockaded woodpecker.

In 1939 President Franklin D. Roosevelt created Piedmont NWR by executive order. The land was substantially different than it now appears. Cleared and planted by settlers who grew cotton as their cash crop, the land was mostly abandoned by 1939 because of decreasing cotton prices, boll weevil infestations, and

Directions

Take I-75 South to Exit 186, Juliette Road/Tift College Drive. Turn left on Juliette Road, at the end of the ramp. After crossing a bridge and passing through East Juliette, the road becomes Juliette-Round Oak Road. At 11.8 miles bear left at the Piedmont NWR sign. The road to the right goes to Jarrell Plantation. In 5.3 miles turn left on a paved road (designated GA 262 on maps but not on the road). After 0.8 miles the road to the visitor center bears right, and the road to the left continues to the trailhead at 1.3 miles.

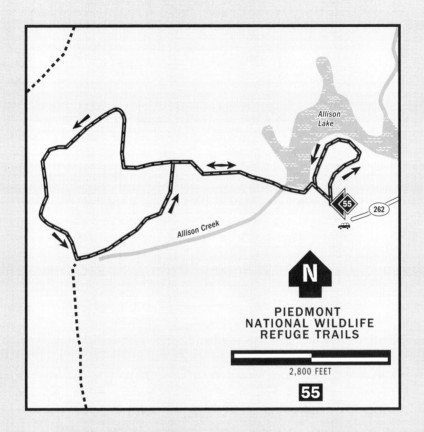

**PIEDMONT
NATIONAL WILDLIFE
REFUGE TRAILS**

2,800 FEET

55

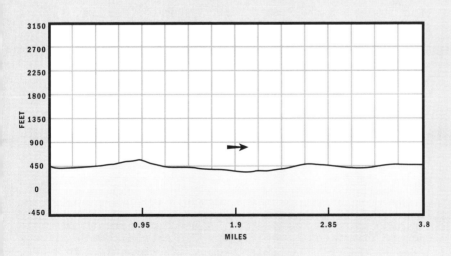

the Great Depression. The biggest problem facing the newly created refuge was erosion—the land was almost completely barren.

Today, thanks to more than 60 years of effective management by the U.S. Fish & Wildlife Service, and Mother Nature, the refuge is returning to a more natural state. The symbol of this regeneration is the red-cockaded woodpecker. The "red" in the bird's name refers to a small patch of color on either side of the bird's head that appears during mating season and territorial battles. The woodpecker is black and white with a large white cheek surrounded by a black head cap and nape on either side of its head.

Both Red-Cockaded Woodpecker (RCW) Trail and Allison Lake Trail begin behind the kiosk. The RCW heads off to the left, making an easy descent through the woods to a gravel road. Turn right and continue descending to a well-marked left turn at Allison Lake, where the trail enters full sun and begins to cross the earthen dam that forms the lake. In the center of the dam, slanted cement sides lead to a flat, wide spillway that you have to cross but may make the trail impassable after a heavy rain when the spillway has running water. Continue on the gravel road to the marked entrance to RCW Trail on the left at 0.3 miles.

Almost immediately you enter a typical Southeastern shortleaf pine second-growth forest that is one of the woodpecker's habitats. Although this bird prefers mature pines infected with red heart fungus, it can be attracted to healthy, younger-growth trees with a little help. The Wildlife Service produces habitat by using artificial inserts, essentially creating a cavity in the pine. The birds nest in these cavities carved in living trees; you'll easily spot the nests by the sap running from them. It is believed that the woodpeckers use the sap to defend against predators such as the rat snake. Trees with inserts are marked with a white circle at the base.

A wooden bench at 0.6 miles marks the start of the loop trail. Turn right and begin a descent to a wooden bridge over a small creek. After the creek the trail bears right and rises to a small knob. On sunny summer days, the area has a number of butterflies, including the tiger swallowtail, viceroy, and zebra. At 1 mile, after the footpath curves left, a gravel road heads off to the right. Just past the road, the trail begins climbing to its highest point.

Begin an extended easy downhill over the next 0.6 miles. Just after beginning the descent, you'll reach a large field with a widely spread group of pines, clearly marked at the base with a ring of white paint. The cavities created by the Wildlife Service attract the woodpeckers and creatures that compete with them for similar nesting, such as the nocturnal flying squirrel. Just past the field, a rarely used road joins the path on the right.

As the trail begins to parallel a creek, the descent eases. Just before you cross the normally dry creek, watch for a red maple with evidence of yellow-bellied sapsuckers. In addition to the maple, this area of hardwoods includes tulip poplar, sweetgum, and a variety of oak. Finally, at 1.8 miles, the trail reaches Allison Creek and a forested wetland that appeared to be fairly active. As the trail began its climb back to the start of the loop, we noted an active beaver den. The trail also lost its definition, but follow the "well-worn trail" principle to return to the bench where the loop started, at 2.3 miles. Turn right and return to the trailhead kiosk.

On the fall day on which we visited Piedmont Wildlife Refuge, Allison Lake Loop was packed with all kinds of animals, from common to exotic. Bring your binoculars and be prepared to spend some quiet time in a blind when walking this trail that begins behind the trailhead kiosk to the right. The trail is interpreted, so pick up a brochure at the kiosk. The numbers in the brochure correspond to those on signs bearing symbols resembling a hiker's boot print. Unlike RCW Trail, Allison Lake Loop is mostly shaded, except for a portion by the lakeshore. At the start, shortleaf pines dominate, but as the trail descends the knob, the number of hardwoods increases.

Initially, the pathway descends, crossing a number of normally dry creek beds, then it rises to a knob. A flash of yellow in the pines led us to believe a pine warbler was out looking for insects. Descending the knob the trail falls to the lake, eventually turning left and running parallel to but above the lakeshore. On the far side of the water, we spotted deer and wild turkey that were surprisingly close to one another. The plaintive call of the mourning dove and the rat-a-tat-tat of a woodpecker added to the excitement.

Finally, on the approach to the lake, we realized we were in for a treat. A kingfisher watched the water for fish. On the far side of the shore, a snowy egret waded among the grass, not bothering a line of turtles sunning on a submerged branch. At 3.4 miles a blind for watching waterfowl juts out into Allison Lake.

NEARBY ATTRACTIONS

The Whistle Stop Café in Juliette, Georgia, is well known for its fried green tomatoes. It was featured in the film of that name starring Jessica Tandy and Kathy Bates in 1991. Phone (478) 994-3670. Jarrell Plantation is a Georgia State Park featuring an interpreted tour of an 18th-century Georgia estate. The plantation is open Tuesday through Saturday from 9 a.m. to 5 p.m., and Sunday from 2 p.m. to 5:30 p.m., but is closed Mondays (except holidays) and on Thanksgiving, December 25, and January 1. Also, it is closed Tuesday when it's open on Monday. Phone (478) 986-5172 for more information.

56 SPREWELL BLUFF TRAIL

 KEY AT-A-GLANCE INFORMATION

LENGTH: 3.2 miles

CONFIGURATION: Out-and-back

DIFFICULTY: Easy, except in the area of the double overlook, where it is difficult

SCENERY: Long-distance views of the Flint River

EXPOSURE: Full sun

TRAFFIC: Light

TRAIL SURFACE: Compacted soil

HIKING TIME: 1.5 hours

ACCESS: Daily, 7 a.m.–sunset

MAPS: USGS Roland

FACILITIES: Restrooms; picnic tables and grills

SPECIAL COMMENTS: Mostly wide, with only a couple of steep sections, this is a great trail to enjoy with the family.

UTM Trailhead Coordinates

UTM Zone (NAD27) 16S

Easting 0735751

Northing 3637628

IN BRIEF

This Georgia State Park hiking trail climbs to a high view of the Flint River, then follows the river past the base of Sprewell Bluff to a natural dam.

DESCRIPTION

Wide, clear, and fast-flowing at Sprewell Bluffs State Park, the Flint River begins as runoff from Atlanta's Hartsfield-Jackson Airport. This was the heart of Creek territory and near the homesite of Benjamin Hawkins, superintendent of Indian Affairs for the Southeast at the start of the 19th century. For more than 20 years, Hawkins represented the United States to the Creek and supervised the representatives to the other Native American nations. Hawkins is credited with the saying, "God willing and the Creek don't rise," which had nothing to do with a stream overflowing its banks but the perception that the Creek were warlike. Hawkins witnessed the devastation brought on by the war with the Red Sticks, a violent faction of the Creek tribe, in 1813 and

----

Directions ⟶

Take I-75 South, Exit 201 (GA 36/Barnesville). Turn right at the end of the ramp and travel 11.4 miles, where GA 36 Bypass heads off to the right. Continue on this road 1.1 miles and turn left on US 7/341. Travel 3.1 miles and turn right on GA 36. Travel 15.5 miles; GA 36 turns right in downtown Thomaston. Continue on GA 36 1.3 miles, where it bears right and merges with GA 74. In 4.2 miles turn left on Old Alabama Road at the brown sign for Sprewell Bluff. The gated entrance to the park comes in 5.4 miles, where you pay the entrance fee ($3). Travel 1.1 miles farther, to the picnic area on the banks of the Flint River.

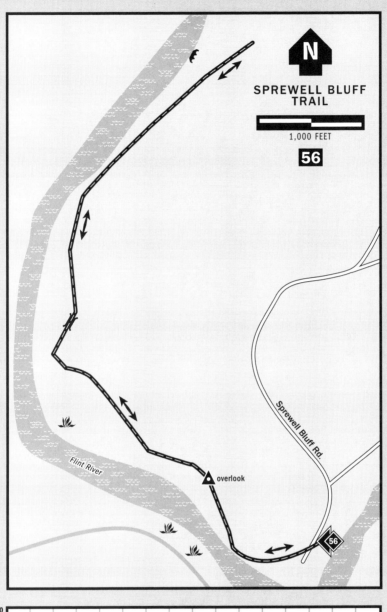

SPREWELL BLUFF
TRAIL

1,000 FEET

56

Flint River

overlook

Sprewell Bluff Rd.

56

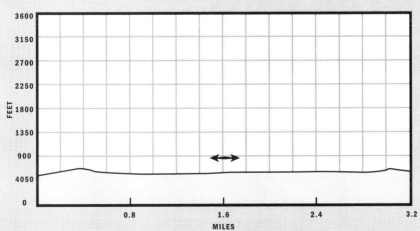

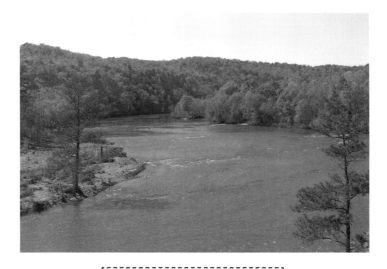

1814. In the same way that the Cherokee were forced west on the Trail of Tears, the Creek were forcibly evicted from their homeland after the Treaty of Indian Springs (1825).

From the parking area, look just in front of the tree line for the restrooms on the right. To the left of the structure is the trailhead, with a brown kiosk with a shingle roof. Beginning as a dirt road, the trail easily rises through an oak, maple, elm, and American beech forest. Quickly a path comes off to the right, but continue straight ahead 0.4 miles, where double overlooks give you a stunning view of the Flint River basin and nearby watershed. As you come off the second overlook, the road splits. Bear left, and the road follows a ridge to a moderately steep but short drop to the river's floodplain.

As you move farther from the rocky precipice, the floodplain widens and the diversity of the forest increases as river birch, dogwood, and ash join the other hardwoods. On the left, a number of trails lead down to the water for fishing. As the trail heads upriver, it begins to move away from the Flint; you can no longer hear the river at 0.7 miles. There is a trailhead kiosk a short distance later. At the kiosk a gravel road heads off to the right and climbs into the Flint River watershed, but continue around the curve to the left, which dips, then rises and curves right to reach a wooden restroom with a fiberglass roof.

As the trail turns left, it once again dips into a moist, bog-like area of the floodplain of the Flint River, then rises to a low ridge and turns right. Less than 0.1 mile later, the trail bears right, turning inland to a three-way intersection at 0.9 miles. Turn left and cross a creek in a culvert through an oak, loblolly pine, and longleaf pine forest. After crossing the creek, the path turns left again and falls to a marshy area that may be difficult to cross after a heavy rain. Just beyond this, the trail joins the riverbank and turns right. As you approach the end of the

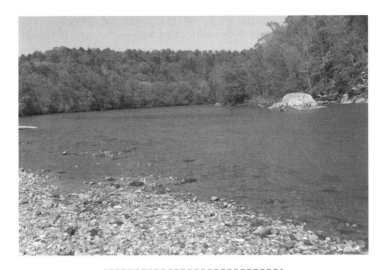

View of Flint River at the trailhead

trail, the sound of the water flowing over the natural dam becomes very loud.

Heading off to the left at 1.5 miles, a side trail allows you to explore a sandy area and catch some good riverside views. Return to the main trail, turn left, and continue a few steps to a second viewing area with a better view of the dam, which is actually a series of rocks that seems to form a narrow shoal. The trail continues down to a clearly marked end just a few steps past the second viewing area. At this point, turn around and retrace your steps to the double overlook.

After the second overlook, watch for a trail that heads off to the right and makes a moderate-to-difficult descent to the Flint River floodplain. Turn left and follow the riverbank. Sprewell Bluff is on the opposite side of the Flint River, rising 150 feet above the river. There are a number of rock outcroppings above the bank. The trail continues to a sign alerting people to the possibility of rapidly rising water. Return along the riverbank to your car.

NEARBY ATTRACTIONS

One of the best-known and oldest attractions in Georgia is Callaway Gardens, 22 miles west of Sprewell Bluffs State Park. In addition to a wide variety of accommodations and restaurants, Callaway offers world-class golf and some surprisingly interesting attractions. As you leave the park, turn left on Roland Road. At 2.1 miles, turn right on GA 36. Travel 12.1 miles to GA 41, then turn right and travel 5.7 miles, turning left on GA 190. In 11 miles GA 354 heads off to the right. Take this road 4 miles to the entrance to Callaway Gardens on the left.

57 STARRS MILL TRAIL

KEY AT-A-GLANCE INFORMATION

LENGTH: 1.5 miles

CONFIGURATION: Out-and-back

DIFFICULTY: Easy

SCENERY: Red mill and dam, river views

EXPOSURE: Full sun

TRAFFIC: Light

TRAIL SURFACE: Gravel road

HIKING TIME: 45 minutes

ACCESS: October–March: daily, 6:30 a.m.–6 p.m.; April–September: daily, 6:30 a.m.–8:30 p.m.

MAPS: USGS Senoia

FACILITIES: None

SPECIAL COMMENTS: No bodily contact with the water allowed. The mill is occasionally used as a filming location for movies and local TV. It was featured in *Sweet Home Alabama*, a 2002 film starring Reese Witherspoon. The dark red mill with a white porch and white trim was the glassworks shop where Josh Lucas's character also served food.

IN BRIEF

Explore Starrs Mill, the pond that powers the mill, and Whitewater Creek, and view a swamp at the north end of Starrs Mill Pond.

DESCRIPTION

Starrs Mill is the picturesque centerpiece of this 16-acre Fayette County Park. Purchased by the county water system in February 1991, the park contains both Starrs Mill and Starrs Mill Pond, which the county intends to use as a water source as demand increases.

From the small gravel parking lot, walk toward the mill. Before the steps to the porch, there is a ramp made of concrete blocks. Follow this down to Whitewater Creek, below the dam. When water levels are low, a small shoal extends almost entirely across the creek and affords a good place to see both the dam and the mill. Return to the mill's porch steps from the shoal. Built on aboveground pilings, the millworks were housed underneath the mill, but the grinding was done in the mill itself. A door on the river side of the mill allowed access to the millworks.

Many years ago, mills such as this were the focal point in rural areas nationwide. Farmers would bring their grains to be ground

UTM Trailhead Coordinates

UTM Zone (NAD27)   16S

Easting   0731885

Northing   3690353

Directions

From Atlanta take I-85 South to Exit 41, Moreland/Newnan. Turn right on Alternate US 27 and travel 0.4 miles to GA 16. Turn right and travel 15.3 miles to GA 74. Turn left on GA 74/85 and continue for 3 miles. At a traffic light, GA 74 turns left. Continue straight ahead on GA 85. Continue 0.3 miles after the light and turn left at Whitewater Way (gravel road). Turn right at 0.1 mile to enter the park.

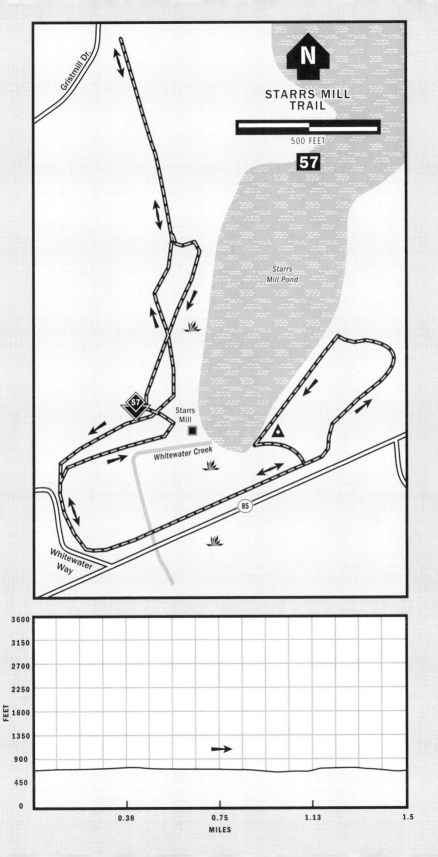

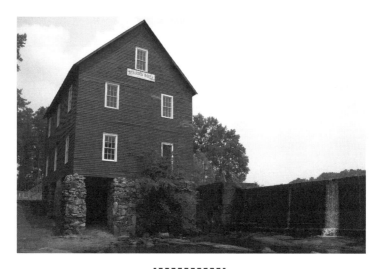

Starr's Mill

(or cracked: hence, the term cracker). Mills were places to exchange political views and gossip and normally included a post office or small grocery. Many times, towns would spring up around mills, as did the town of Starrs Mill.

Be careful climbing the steps to the mill's porch—even a casual inspection shows signs of rot. As you reach the top of the stairs, peek inside the window for a look at the grinding apparatus in the center of the floor. Continue on and exit down the front of the porch, returning to the gravel road. Past the mill is an outbuilding, around which the road curves as it rises. Once around the building, follow the road to a T-intersection and turn left.

On your right is an extensive marshland that makes up the upper reaches of Starrs Mill Pond. In the distance you'll probably see at least a few of the larger common swamp birds, including egrets, herons, and mourning doves. As the road begins to rise, a No Trespassing sign indicates the park boundary. Turn around and return to the T-intersection, then continue straight ahead. As the road curves to the right, it returns to the lakeshore.

Fishing is a popular pastime at this pond, and anglers normally park at least a couple of cars along the road. The clear land at the water's edge offers an excellent view of the entire lake. During late fall and early spring, migratory birds, especially geese, visit the pond. Return via the gravel road to Starrs Mill parking lot. From the lot walk past the picnic tables down to the river's edge and follow it, walking away from the mill.

Looking down Whitewater Creek, notice the luxuriant growth along the banks. These vegetated borders are known as the riparian zones, and the full, lush growth is indicative of both a healthy river and clean water. The plants hold the banks in place, even during high water, and provide nesting grounds for amphibians and insects and shelter for small animals. As you walk along the river it suddenly makes a 90-degree turn and flows toward the bridge over GA 85. At this long-distance view, notice that the creek's riparian zones continue as far as the eye can see.

Return to the gravel road and follow it as it curves to the left to the entrance of the park at Waterfall Way. Turn left, continue to GA 85, and turn left again. Walk over the bridge across Whitewater Creek and turn left down a dirt driveway.

Continue walking along the creek side, toward the dam. After heavy rainfalls the size of the water flow over the dam enhances photographs of the mill. Once past the dam, you'll see the lake, and on windless days the mill reflects in the millpond. Photographers should get here before sunrise to capture the mill in the morning light. Mid-November is especially beautiful, thanks to the autumn colors of the maple trees behind the mill.

As you walk along the lakeshore, the path reaches the low rise that forms the swamp and becomes overgrown. Turn right and continue to the road embankment, then turn right again and return to the gravel driveway. Climb to GA 85, turn right, and return to the parking lot via Waterfall Way.

NEARBY ATTRACTIONS

Dauset Trails in Jackson features hiking, biking, and horseback trails. It is open Monday through Saturday from 9 a.m. to 5 p.m., and Sunday from noon to 5 p.m. Call (770) 775-6798 for more information.

58 SWEETWATER HISTORIC (RED) AND YELLOW TRAIL

KEY AT-A-GLANCE INFORMATION

LENGTH: 5.7 miles

CONFIGURATION: Double loop

DIFFICULTY: Moderate, except for the portion between Sweetwater Mill and the falls, which is difficult

SCENERY: Scenic views of Sweetwater Creek, falls, historic mill

EXPOSURE: Full sun to part shade along the riverbanks, mostly shaded elsewhere

TRAFFIC: Heavy on the trail to the mill, moderate elsewhere

TRAIL SURFACE: Compacted soil

HIKING TIME: 4 hours

ACCESS: Park hours: Daily, 7 a.m.–10 p.m.; trails close at dark.

MAPS: USGS Austell, Mableton, Campbellton, Ben Hill

FACILITIES: Restrooms, picnic areas, pavilions

SPECIAL COMMENTS: Sweetwater Creek is one of the largest tributaries of the Chattahoochee River. The confluence of these two rivers is only a couple of miles from the mill.

UTM Trailhead Coordinates

UTM Zone (NAD27) 16S

Easting 0719697

Northing 3737140

IN BRIEF

The Red, or Historic, Trail follows an old road through the historic city of New Manchester to Sweetwater Mill then continues to an over-look of Sweetwater Creek falls. The Yellow Trail crosses the river and climbs into the watershed before returning along the river.

DESCRIPTION

After purchasing this land in 1845, former Georgia governor Charles McDonald began construction on Sweetwater Manufacturing Company in 1846. Sweetwater began producing thread, yarn, and cloth three years later. The mill was taller than any building in nearby Atlanta when completed. In 1857 Sweetwater was reorganized as the New Manchester Manufacturing Company, the name it retained until it was destroyed by Union troops on July 9, 1864.

From the trailhead kiosk at the east end of the parking lot, Sweetwater Historic (Red) Trail descends gradually to Sweetwater Creek, turning right at 0.2 miles and following the curves of the bank of Sweetwater Creek. The trail is a

---

Directions

Take I-20 West to Exit 44, GA 6/Thorton Road/Austell. As you come to the end of the ramp, stay in the right-hand left-turn lane. After turning on Thorton Road, travel 0.1 mile and make a right on Blair's Bridge Road, at the Toyota dealership. At 2.4 miles turn left on Mount Vernon Road. This road enters Sweetwater Park at 0.6 miles. Continue 1.4 miles to the signed turn to the visitor center. Immediately after the turn, you'll reach a pay booth on the left. If it is open, pay the $3 parking fee; otherwise, pay at any one of the self-service stations throughout the park. Continue down this road to the parking lot.

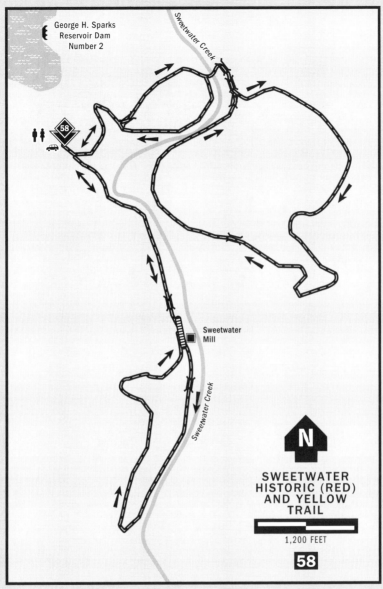

George H. Sparks
Reservoir Dam
Number 2

Sweetwater Creek

58

Sweetwater
Mill

Sweetwater Creek

N

SWEETWATER
HISTORIC (RED)
AND YELLOW
TRAIL

1,200 FEET

58

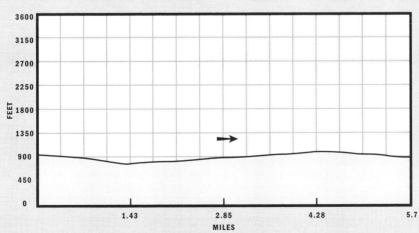

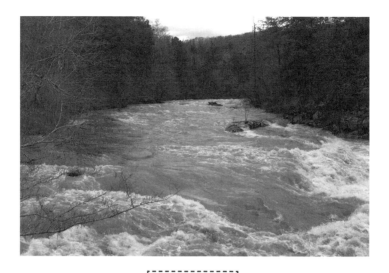

Sweetwater Falls

wide, level gravel road through a forest of American beech, white oak, loblolly pine, and sweetgum. Watch for a large square indentation on the right and an interpretive sign on the left that tells the story of New Manchester. Here Nathaniel Humphries ran the company store that contained a post office and possibly a shoe-manufacturing operation during the Civil War. On the left is the start of the millrace that ends at Sweetwater Manufacturing. Almost immediately a wooden bridge allows you to cross the millrace and explore what is now a man-made island. Return to the main trail and continue to the left. At the end of the island, the spillway is now used to divert the water from the mill in an attempt to preserve it.

A wooden walkway before the mill on the left gives you an up-close look at the power room of Sweetwater Mill at 0.6 miles. Notice that the old bed of the millrace makes a 90-degree turn between the platform and the closest end of the building. Water from Sweetwater Creek coursing through the millrace followed this curve into the power room, where it would turn a wheel, generating power. Machinery in the middle room wove the thread, yarn, and fabric, which was stored at the far end of the building to be transported to Atlanta.

The Sweetwater Blue Trail continues straight, but the Sweetwater Historic (Red) Trail turns left after passing the mill and descends on a set of wooden steps, quickly coming to the end of the boardwalk. From this point to Sweetwater Falls, we consider this trail difficult because there are multiple trail-narrowing rock outcrops, and the trail is rocky and heavily rooted. A chain railing carries hikers across a particularly difficult area at 0.8 miles after which one reaches a wooden bridge and an overlook. Just over a mile into the hike, a series of rock outcrops narrows the path. As the trail curves right, into a cove, a massive 25-foot boulder seems to block the way, but wooden steps allow trekkers to scale the rock.

Hikers making it to the top of the rock are rewarded with an excellent view from the first of two platforms over the next 0.1 mile. Continue to the second platform for a superb view of Sweetwater Falls. As you leave the platform, climb the steps straight ahead and follow the Sweetwater Blue Trail to return to the mill. At the mill take the Sweetwater Historic (Red) Trail and return to the trailhead. Just before the starting point, watch for a side trail on the right with a yellow blaze and a brown hiking sign. After turning right and crossing a gravel road, the Sweetwater Yellow Trail curves to the left.

The pathway begins a long, easy descent into a river valley, making a U-turn near a paved park road and running alongside a creek to a wooden bridge. Turn left and cross the bridge; the trail straight ahead is the return trail. Although this footpath continues straight, it is frequently too muddy to traverse, so turn left on a gravel road at 2.8 miles. Turn right at the next road and follow this to Ferguson's Bridge. Technically known as an M-6 bridge, this modern structure was in use from 1958 until 1983. An antebellum structure that spanned the river in about the same place was used to haul bricks and lumber for the mill from the far side of the river.

After crossing the bridge, walk down the steps to the right. The footpath winds along the riverbank and comes to a wooden bridge. Shortly after the bridge, 3.2 miles into the hike, turn left on the Sweetwater Yellow Trail and begin an extended climb into the watershed of Sweetwater Creek. Over the next 0.8 miles the trail rises some 300 feet in full sun. Watch for a yellow-topped post on the left and three consecutively blazed trees. The signs are there to ensure you don't turn on the historic road, which heads off to the left. Continue straight on the Sweetwater Yellow Trail to a right turn marked by a double blaze.

Still climbing, the Sweetwater Yellow Trail turns left at 3.8 miles, and there is a scenic view less than 0.1 mile later, after a marked right-hand turn. As the trail continues around to the right, it comes to a bench, then bears left, beginning to run along a creek bed as it descends. In an area of rock outcroppings and cascades, the trail rock-hops across the stream, crossing back on a bridge a little later. Reaching the riverbank the trail curves right and easily climbs back to the loop's start. Retrace your steps to Ferguson Bridge, but turn left after the crossing. Following the bank of the river, the trail returns you to the bridge near the start of the Sweetwater Yellow Trail.

NEARBY ATTRACTIONS

George Sparks Reservoir is a great place to take the kids fishing for bream, crappie, catfish, and an occasional bass. The Georgia Department of Natural Resources, which manages the 215-acre reservoir, has added brush along the banks to make them fish-friendly. You can also rent an electric-powered boat for an offshore adventure.

59 SWEETWATER NONGAME WILDLIFE TRAILS

KEY AT-A-GLANCE INFORMATION

LENGTH: 5.1 miles

CONFIGURATION: Loop

DIFFICULTY: Moderate

SCENERY: Creekside views, long-distance views into a river gorge, lake, remains of a cotton mill, and waterfalls

EXPOSURE: Mostly shaded, except during the first mile and in the vicinity of the river

TRAFFIC: Moderate, except in the vicinity of the cotton mill and falls, where it is heavy

TRAIL SURFACE: Gravel roads, historic roads, and compacted dirt

HIKING TIME: 3 hours

ACCESS: Open daylight hours

MAPS: Available at visitor center; USGS Austell, Mableton, Ben Hill, Campbellton

FACILITIES: Restrooms, picnic tables with grills

SPECIAL COMMENTS: Arrive at this trail early in the morning to see the most wildlife.

UTM Trailhead Coordinates

UTM Zone (NAD27) 16S

Easting   0719574

Northing   3737091

IN BRIEF

This deep-woods experience is only a few minutes west of downtown Atlanta. Hikers on the Nongame Wildlife Trails frequently see deer, wild turkey, and other large animals.

DESCRIPTION

Sweetwater Nongame Wildlife Trails, known as Sweetwater White and Sweetwater Blue, begin as a gravel road, on the right side of the visitor center as you face the building. Almost immediately, the return loop joins the trail from the left. Over the first 1.3 miles, the well-marked treadway follows gravel roads and occasionally enters the woods. Within the picnic area, Sweetwater White crosses two paved roads, quickly reentering forest each time, and becoming a gravel road at 0.6 miles. At a three-way intersection, the trail bears left at 0.8 miles. For no apparent reason, the trail makes a left-hand jog, then turns almost immediately to the right, into the woods, at 1.2 miles. It returns to a dirt road a little farther along in the hike. At the top of a knoll, the trail makes a right turn at a four-way intersection, follows the ridge 0.3 miles, then

---

Directions ⟶

Take I-20 West to Exit 44, GA 6/Thorton Road/Austell. As you come to the end of the ramp, stay in the right-hand left-turn lane. Travel 0.1 mile on Thorton Road and make a right on Blair's Bridge Road, at the Toyota dealership. At 2.4 miles turn left on Mount Vernon Road. This road enters Sweetwater Park at 0.6 miles. Continue 1.4 miles to the signed turn to the visitor center. Immediately after the turn, there is a pay booth. If it is open, pay the $3 parking fee; otherwise, pay at any one of the self-service stations throughout the park. Continue down this road to the parking lot.

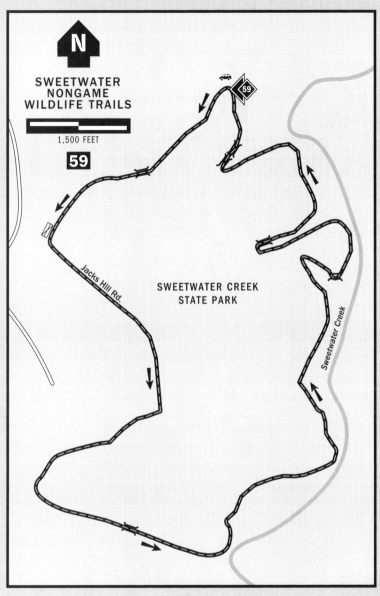

SWEETWATER
NONGAME
WILDLIFE TRAILS

1,500 FEET

59

SWEETWATER CREEK
STATE PARK

Jacks Hill Rd.

Sweetwater Creek

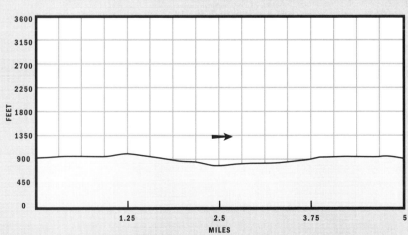

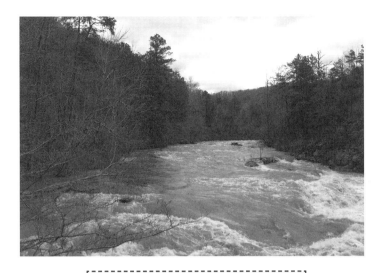

Sweetwater Creek Falls at the Brevard Fault Line

turns right again and begins a dramatic easy-to-moderate descent into the Sweetwater Creek river valley.

Almost immediately the valley on the right drops off, the sides become steep, and the area is filled with a diverse, second-growth oak and American beech forest. As the road follows the curve of the mountain to the left, there is a scenic view on the right of a lake formed by a dammed creek. The trail continues wrapping around the mountain, still descending as it begins to parallel the lakeshore. After the pathway levels, it turns right and begins crossing the earthen dam to a set of long wooden steps on the left that carry you down to a streamside trail. Before descending these steps, spend a few minutes watching for large waterfowl that visit the lake. The path traverses moist, fern-covered soil to a double bridge at 2 miles.

After the bridge the trail follows a historic road past a massive granite boulder that signifies a change—the number of rock outcroppings begins to increase, as does the number and size of boulders in the creek bed. Near 2.4 miles the treadway bears left and comes out at a park bench facing the normally loud Sweetwater Creek, which at this point is completing a rapid descent (a 60-foot drop in just over 0.5 miles) through the fractured and sheared rock of the Brevard Fault zone. The trail briefly joins Sweetwater Creek before it moves slightly inland and up, climbing a massive rock outcropping along the river, where the creek crashes over a series of boulders. After climbing around the outcrop, the trail returns to run along the creek bank, offering good long-distance views into the gorge formed by the hills on either side of the creek. Step across a rivulet at 2.7 miles, then climb the wooden steps at 3 miles for an excellent view of the falls, where the river tumbles through a series of cascades.

After the steps Sweetwater White crosses a rocky area and a bridge; then it reaches a T-intersection with Sweetwater Blue at a second set of stairs. Turn right and descend to the overlook that marks the end of both the Sweetwater Historic (Red) Trail (see page 258) and the Sweetwater Blue Trail. Once again you'll find good scenic views into the gorge that was formed over eons by Sweetwater Creek. From the overlook, turn around and begin climbing the steps, passing Sweetwater White on your left and continuing to the top of a small hill. Still in a diverse hardwood forest, Sweetwater Blue turns right, then follows the curve of the hill as the river comes into view some 100 feet below.

Almost entirely in the forest, Sweetwater Blue is a significantly different trail than Sweetwater White. At 3.5 miles the trail curves sharply inland, exploring a lush cove and tributary of Sweetwater Creek. Watch the trail closely as it joins one of the many historic roads that crosscut these once populated hills. The trail makes a U-turn deep in the cove, and the footpath leaves the road. As you approach the gorge of Sweetwater Creek, the trail curves left, falling easily to the remains of a three-story brick cotton mill that was once the tallest building in the Atlanta area. Sweetwater Manufacturing began production in 1849. Eventually, New Manchester Manufacturing was formed, and Sweetwater became a part of that larger operation. In 1864 the Union cavalry captured the mill and burned it to the ground. For more information on the mill at New Manchester, see Sweetwater Historic (Red) Trail (page 258).

Leaving the mill, turn right; the Red and Blue trails immediately split. Follow the Blue Trail to the left as it rises and moves inland, once again following a gravel road deep into a forested cove. At 4.2 miles the road makes a U-turn in the cove and returns to a winter view of the creek on the right 0.2 miles later. Paralleling the river, but running well away from it, the trail slowly curves left until it makes a hard left on a gravel road at 4.7 miles. This roadway carries you into another cove, turning right to leave the road, crossing a bridge, and turning right again, until the trail reaches the visitor center.

NEARBY ATTRACTIONS

The kids might enjoy a trip to Six Flags after this hike. The park is heavily into roller coaster–style rides, beginning with the traditional roller-coaster rides Great American Scream Machine and the Georgia Cyclone. Other coasters have more contemporary themes, and the newest, Goliath, is a "hypercoaster," which means it's built for speed and airtime. Thunder River and Splashwater Falls are fun water rides. Take I-20 toward Atlanta for 2 miles to Exit 46. Exit at Six Flags and follow the signs. Opening times and prices vary according to the season. Call (770) 948-9290 for more information or visit their Web site at **www.sixflags .com/overgeorgia.**

60 WOLFDEN LOOP: PINE MOUNTAIN TRAIL

KEY AT-A-GLANCE INFORMATION

LENGTH: 6.7 miles

CONFIGURATION: Loop

DIFFICULTY: Moderate

SCENERY: Multiple waterfalls, long-distance view of Georgia's coastal plain from the Beaver Dam Trail

EXPOSURE: Mostly shaded

TRAFFIC: Heavy from the Roadside Park area to the Wolf's Den, moderate elsewhere

TRAIL SURFACE: Compacted soil

HIKING TIME: 4 hours

ACCESS: Open year-round

MAPS: 2 maps available at the park office for a fee that goes to support the Pine Mountain Trail Association; USGS Shiloh

FACILITIES: No facilities on the trail or in the parking areas

SPECIAL COMMENTS: Native azalea, dogwood, rhododendron, and mountain laurel bloom in April and May; central Georgia's leaves change well into November.

UTM Trailhead Coordinates

UTM Zone (NAD27) 16S

Easting 0713391

Northing 3638205

IN BRIEF

Wolfden Loop explores waterfalls along Wolfden Branch and Cascade Branch of Cane Creek then follows a ridge back.

DESCRIPTION

From the east end of the Rocky Point parking area, turn right and climb the steps to immediately enter a second-growth forest that was once part of a farm owned by Franklin D. Roosevelt. The land was donated to Georgia after his death in 1945 at nearby Warm Springs; the state acquired additional land in the area and created Franklin Delano Roosevelt (FDR) State Park. It is the largest state park in the Georgia Department of Natural Resources system.

A scant 0.1 mile into the forest, the blue-blazed Pine Mountain Trail curves right, and the white-blazed Beaver Dam Trail turns left. Follow Beaver Dam Trail. The valley on your right disappears and a steep-sided 200-foot cliff replaces it as the trail follows the curve of the mountain to the right. There are a couple of long-distance scenic views into Georgia's coastal plain as you enter the semiarid conditions on this escarpment. On the south side

Directions

Take I-85 South to Exit 41, GA 14/US 27 Alt. At the end of the ramp, turn left. Follow US 27A as it loops around the courthouse in Greenville at 21 miles, returning to the original road after the courthouse. Turn right on Spring Street (GA 85A). Travel 3.9 miles and turn right on GA 190. The parking area on the right at 3.8 miles is often full on weekends. Travel 2.1 miles to the Rocky Point parking. Back into a space, then walk to the east side of the lot to begin the hike.

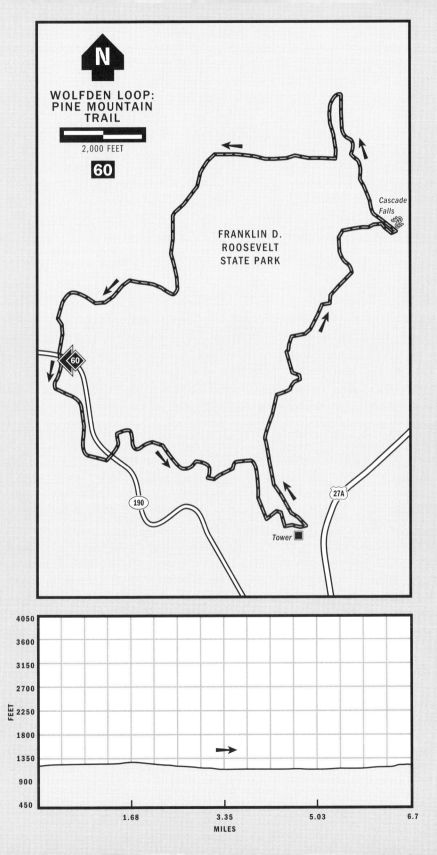

WOLFDEN LOOP:
PINE MOUNTAIN
TRAIL

2,000 FEET

60

FRANKLIN D.
ROOSEVELT
STATE PARK

Cascade
Falls

60

190

27A

Tower

MILES

of the mountain sandy soil fills gaps in the rocky mountainside so rainfall quickly evaporates leaving little moisture for undergrowth. The rocky mountain prevents the trees from growing tall, and the landscape assumes a xenotropic appearance. This is the first and the briefest of the three ecosystems through which the trail passes.

After crossing a historic road, the trail curves left and leaves the south-facing mountainside. Undergrowth and tree size begin increasing. By the time the trail reaches GA 190 (at 0.6 miles), the forest has returned to the transitional pine of the Georgia piedmont. Just before 1 mile, the number of hardwoods begins to increase, marking the second ecosystem. Soil moisture is higher in part because of the higher humus content. Trees with full crowns moderate the heat of the sun, making the forest cooler and increasing the moisture content of the soil. Point out to the kids in the group that there are many different types of trees, not just pine. One species worth noting is the chestnut oak, also called American chestnut, which can be found near the trail in this area. Watch for unusually large acorns that look like chestnuts; they range from 1 to 1.5 inches in length and are about 1 inch in diameter and have leaves that are up to 6 inches long with rounded (crenate) edges.

Following a short pine blowdown, watch on the left side for a beaver dam that gives the trail its name. As the lake formed by the dam comes to an end, the trail curves left and parallels Pine Mountain Trail to return to the start of the trail near the WJSP-TV tower. At the registration mailbox and kiosk, Beaver Dam Trail dead-ends into Pine Mountain Trail. According to Jim Hall, president of the Pine Mountain Trail Association, the site of FDR's farm is near this intersection. The farm included most of the present-day park from this point to Dowdell's Knob.

Turn left and begin an easy descent along the most heavily traveled portion of Wolfden Loop. Wolfden Branch, one of two streams the trail explores, forms on the left of the trail at the bottom of an easy-sloped valley. Mountain laurel consumes the trail at 2.4 miles, and 0.2 miles later the trail emerges at the top of a natural rock wall that drops some 15 feet immediately to the right of the trail. After the wall the trail curves left and descends to Dry Falls, which normally flows only after a rain and marks the start of the third ecosystem. The stream plays a major role in adding moisture to the ecosystem. Soil, even that significantly far from the stream, retains its moisture because of the high humus level. The full crown of trees and the north-facing position of the cove keep the area cooler than the adjacent ridgetops.

Mile marker 22 is in another patch of mountain laurel that consumes the path, and Csonka Falls appears at 3.1 miles. These falls are formed by a large, almost flat rock with the water flowing over its lowest point to drop into a nearly circular pool of clear mountain water. At 0.3 miles after Csonka Falls, the trail becomes a muddy morass at the appropriately name Slippery Rock Falls. Following the falls, the trail turns and rises—watch for the double blaze indicating the turn. A short trail to Bumblebee Ridge campsite heads off to the left at 3.5 miles.

Wolfden Loop crosses the stream again then begins the moderate climb up Cascade Branch. Just past mile marker 21, Cascade Falls comes into view.

One of FDR's favorite sites on his farm, Cascade Falls flows in from the right side, dropping in a series of 10 to 15 cascades. The stream then turns and drops in three or four falls to a flat rock, culminating in a single four-foot drop. Twenty feet to the right of the falls is a plaque in memory of Michael Preston Brown, a charter member of the Pine Mountain Trail Association. Leaving the falls, the trail turns left and ascends the small, handmade rock steps that lead to the Wolfden, a sheer rock wall with an overhang at the bottom. Climbing away from the Wolfden, the trail runs adjacent to a steep-sided drop on the left. Both tree size and the number of boulders begin to increase.

Once again the trail dips to Wolfden Branch, crosses it, then rises to a rock formation commonly known as a fat man's squeeze. Old Sawmill campsite is down a short trail on the left, which means Ferney, the 14-foot-circumference pine tree that is almost directly on the trail, is coming up. Other names for the massive tree are Big Pine and Old Pine. A dam on the right at 4.4 miles indicates we are about to leave the cove.

As the footpath makes a lazy U-turn, it begins a moderate-to-difficult climb to the top of Hogback Mountain. Almost as soon as you begin this climb, the undergrowth and tree diversity lessens and the number of pine trees increase, but the forest is still majority hardwood. Mile marker 20 marks a curve to the right where the climb eases significantly. At 5.7 miles the climb abates, having risen a total of 300 feet in 1.3 miles. From this point on, the path falls and rises at an easy-to-moderate grade back to the Rocky Point parking area.

NEARBY ATTRACTIONS

Warm Springs is the site of the Little White House, rich with the history of President Franklin D. Roosevelt. The Georgia State Park is open daily, 9 a.m. to 4:45 p.m., except Thanksgiving, December 25, and January 1. Phone (706) 655-5870 for more information.

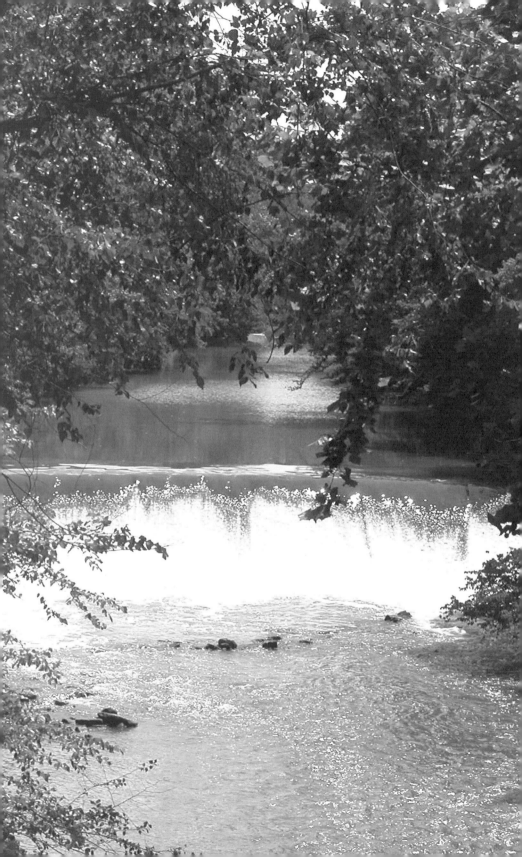

60 HIKES
WITHIN 60 MILES

ATLANTA
INCLUDING
MARIETTA, LAWRENCEVILLE, AND PEACHTREE CITY

APPENDIXES
AND INDEX

APPENDIX A:
HIKING STORES

Bass Pro Shops
Outdoor World
www.basspro.com
5900 Sugarloaf Parkway
Lawrenceville, GA 30043
(678) 847-5500

Bargain Barn
www.bargainbarn.com
3622 Camp Road
Jasper, GA 30143
(706) 253-WHOA
(877) 337-WHOA

Dick's Sporting Goods
www.dickssportinggoods.com

Atlanta
Lenox Marketplace
3535 Peachtree Road
Atlanta, GA 30326 (404) 267-0200

Buford
Mall of Georgia
3333 Buford Drive
Buford, GA 30519
(678) 482-1200

Kennesaw
Town Center
691 Ernest W. Barrett Parkway
Kennesaw, GA 30144
(770) 281-0200

High Country Outfitters
www.highcountryoutfitters.com
3906 Roswell Road NE
Atlanta, GA 30342
(404) 814-0999

5165 Peachtree Parkway NW
Norcross, GA 30092
(770) 409-4908

Hit The Trail
www.hitthetrailonline.com
10 Lagrange Street
Newnan, GA 30263
(770) 253-2241

Mountain Crossings at Walesi-yi
www.mountaincrossings.com
9710 Gainesville Highway
Blairsville, GA 30512
(706) 745-6095

North Georgia Mountain Outfitters
www.hikenorthgeorgia.com
1215 Industrial Boulevard
East Ellijay, GA 30540
(706) 698-HIKE

REI
www.rei.com

Atlanta
1800 Northeast Expressway NE
Atlanta, GA 30329
(404) 633-6508

Kennesaw
740 Barrett Parkway, Suite 450
Kennesaw, GA 30144
(770) 425-4480

Perimeter
1165 Perimeter Center West, Suite 200
Atlanta, GA 30338
(770) 901-9200

APPENDIX A:
HIKING STORES [CONTINUED]

REI (*continued*)
Buford
1600 Mall of Georgia Boulevard, Suite 800
Buford, GA 30519
(770) 831-0676

The Outside World
www.theoutsideworld.net
471 Quill Drive
Dawsonville, GA 30534
(706) 265-4500

APPENDIX B:
HIKING CLUBS

Pine Mountain Trail Association
www.pinemountaintrail.org

Benton MacKaye Trail Association
www.bmta.org

The Georgia Appalachian Trail Club
www.georgia-atclub.org

Atlanta Single Hikers
http://www.atlantasinglehikers.com/

Fun Hikes
www.funhikes.com

INDEX

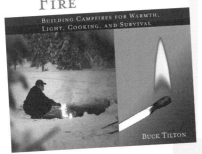
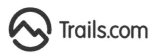
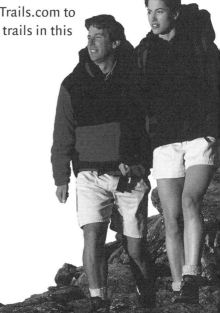

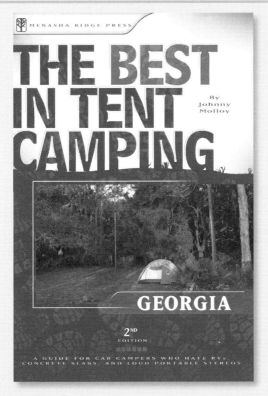

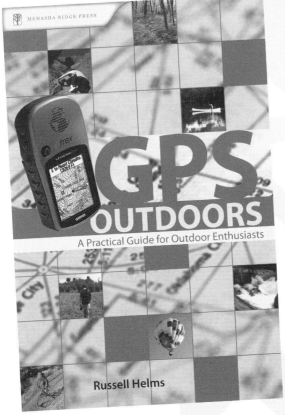

GPS OUTDOORS

by Russell Helms
ISBN 10: 0-89732-967-8
ISBN 13: 978-0-89732-967-5
$10.95
120pages

Whether you're a hiker on a weekend trip through the Great Smokies, a backpacker cruising the Continental Divide Trail, a mountain biker kicking up dust in Moab, a paddler running the Lewis and Clark bicentennial route, or a climber pre-scouting the routes up Mount Shasta, a simple handheld GPS unit is fun, useful, and can even be a lifesaver.

AMERICAN HIKING SOCIETY

Because you **hike.**

We're with you every step of the way

American Hiking Society gives voice to the more than 75 million Americans who hike and is the only national organization that promotes and protects foot trails, the natural areas that surround them and the hiking experience. Our work is inspiring and challenging, and is built on three pillars:

Volunteerism and Stewardship: We organize and coordinate nationally recognized programs – including Volunteer Vacations, National Trails Day® and the National Trails Fund –that help keep our trails open, safe and enjoyable.

Policy and Advocacy: We work with Congress and federal agencies to ensure funding for trails, the preservation of natural areas, and the protection of the hiking experience.

Outreach and Education: We expand and support the national constituency of hikers through outreach and education as well as partnerships with other recreation and conservation organizations.

Join us in our efforts. Become an American Hiking Society member today!

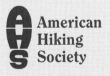

American Hiking Society

1422 Fenwick Lane · Silver Spring, MD 20910 · (301) 565-6704
www.AmericanHiking.org · info@AmericanHiking.org

DEAR CUSTOMERS AND FRIENDS,

SUPPORTING YOUR INTEREST IN OUTDOOR ADVENTURE, travel, and an active lifestyle is central to our operations, from the authors we choose to the locations we detail to the way we design our books. Menasha Ridge Press was incorporated in 1982 by a group of veteran outdoorsmen and professional outfitters. For 25 years now, we've specialized in creating books that benefit the outdoors enthusiast.

Almost immediately, Menasha Ridge Press earned a reputation for revolutionizing outdoors- and travel-guidebook publishing. For such activities as canoeing, kayaking, hiking, backpacking, and mountain biking, we established new standards of quality that transformed the whole genre, resulting in outdoor-recreation guides of great sophistication and solid content. Menasha Ridge continues to be outdoor publishing's greatest innovator.

The folks at Menasha Ridge Press are as at home on a white-water river or mountain trail as they are editing a manuscript. The books we build for you are the best they can be, because we're responding to your needs. Plus, we use and depend on them ourselves.

We look forward to seeing you on the river or the trail. If you'd like to contact us directly, join in at www.trekalong.com or visit us at www.menasharidge.com. We thank you for your interest in our books and the natural world around us all.

SAFE TRAVELS,

BOB SEHLINGER
PUBLISHER